15.

Food and People

Proceedings of the British Nutrition Foundation 4th Annual Conference, held at the Royal College of Physicians, London, 29 and 30 June 1982.

FOOD
and
PEOPLE

Edited by

MICHAEL R. TURNER

The British Nutrition Foundation,
London, UK

John Libbey : London

First published 1983 by

John Libbey & Company Limited
80–84 Bondway, London SW8 1SF

© 1983. Copyright. All rights reserved.

Unauthorised duplication contravenes applicable laws.

British Library Cataloguing in Publication Data

British Nutrition Foundation. *Annual Conference*
    (4th : 1982 : London)
    Food and people.
    1. Nutrition — Congresses
    I. Title   II. Turner, M. R.
    613.2   TX345

    ISBN 0-86196-024-6

Phototypeset by Dobbie Typesetting Service, Plymouth, Devon
Printed by Biddles of Guildford, Surrey

Contributors

M. R. Alderson, *Chief Medical Statistician, Office of Population Censuses & Surveys, St. Catherine's House, 10 Kingsway, London WC2B 6JP.*

Sir Kenneth Blaxter, FRS, *Director (1965–1982), The Rowett Research Institute, Greenburn Road, Bucksburn, Aberdeen AB2 9SB.*

Mildred Blaxter, *Lately Medical Research Council Sociologist, MRC Unit of Medical Sociology, Westburn Road, Aberdeen, AB9 2ZE.*

G. Glew, *Head of Catering Department, The Polytechnic, Huddersfield HD1 3DH.*

Juliet Gray, *Science Director, The British Nutrition Foundation, 15 Belgrave Square, London SW1X 8PS.*

Daphne Grose, MBE, *Head of Representation, The Consumers' Association, 14 Buckingham Street, London WC2N 6DS.*

B. Isaacs, *Charles Hayward Professor of Geriatric Medicine, Department of Geriatric Medicine, The University of Birmingham, The Hayward Building, Selly Oak Hospital, Raddlebarn Road, Birmingham B29 6JD.*

S. H. M. King, *Director, J. Walter Thompson Company Limited, 40 Berkeley Square, London W1X 6AD.*

K. A. Last, *District Catering Manager, Manchester Area Health Authority (Teaching), South District, Withington Hospital, Nell Lane, Manchester M20 8LR.*

H. G. Phillips, *Sales and Marketing Division, Ross Foods, Ross House, Grimsby, DN31 3SW.*

J. A. Rice, *Regional Catering Officer, Wessex Regional Health Authority, Highcroft, Winchester, Hants SO22 5DH.*

Sylvia Robert-Sargeant, *Education Director, The British Nutrition Foundation, 15 Belgrave Square, London SW1X 8PS.*

A. Ward, CBE, *Emeritus Professor of Food Science, Procter Department of Food Science, The University, Leeds.*

Acknowledgements

The British Nutrition Foundation is most grateful to everyone who contributed to the success of the Conference of which this book is a record. It is not possible to name the many people who made suggestions for the scientific programme, but their help and ideas were much appreciated.

The Foundation also wishes to express its appreciation to the invited Chairmen, Dr J. Treasure and Professor Alan Ward CBE, and the speakers, whose presentations at the Conference were so stimulating and whose written papers are published in this book.

Preface

This book is a record of the Proceedings of the British Nutrition Foundation's 4th Annual Conference held at the Royal College of Physicians, London in June 1982 under the title *Food and People*. It is multidisciplinary in its concept and brings together ideas and expertise from: social survey research, medical sociology and medical statistics; the agricultural, food manufacturing and catering sectors; consumer interests; and the food and nutritional sciences.

The Conference set out to focus attention on some sociological bases of problems encountered in implementing nutritional policies, and on opportunities that may exist within the catering, food manufacturing and agricultural sectors for influencing dietary intake along the lines indicated in published dietary guidelines for health.

The book divides into three sections. The first section (Chapters 1 to 3) opens with an account of population and health trends, with particular emphasis on social class, poverty and nutrition. It goes on to review trends in food and meal habits and comments on determinants of these trends insofar as these are understood.

The second section (Chapters 4 to 6) explores the position of the consumer and the food manufacturer at a time of rapid change in social attitudes and behaviour, and in the light of developments which have taken place in recent years in the understanding of relationships between nutrition, health and disease. There follows an overview of influences on food production and how farming meets the changing needs of people.

The remainder of the book (Chapters 7 to 11) is devoted to recent trends in catering in schools, hospitals and community services for the elderly, and highlights the scope that exists for developments in institutional catering based on present knowledge of nutrition and health. An overview of catering in the public sector is included which makes some reference to the place of work and the commercial sector, and also indicates ways in which the study and planning of catering operations may be approached. With an increasing proportion of food being eaten out of the home, the influence of the professional caterer on what people eat is rising.

February 1983   Michael R. Turner

Contents

1

The changing population profile: structure, environment, and health

MICHAEL ALDERSON

A. Introduction

The title implies consideration of a wide range of issues; this obviously means that the amount of detail is very limited for any particular topic, necessitating a broad-brush approach to the matter. This chapter is divided into four rather different parts: the first section deals with aspects of demography, presenting a picture of the present population and changes that have occurred in the make-up of the population over the past century; my intention here is to indicate the main aspects of population change that are related to any alteration in the health of the community, and indirectly to aspects of food policy. The second section turns to a wider range of classifying variates that are related to the health of the population, either directly in influencing the risk of disease, or more indirectly through other factors associated with the determinants of disease. Obviously the range of issues that could be discussed under this heading are very great, and therefore those that are likely to be related to nutrition or diet-related diseases have been highlighted, with consideration also of the range of other important variates that contribute to a major part of the known aetiology of diseases. The final two sections deal with those routine sets of statistics that point up the health of the population, or measure the burden of disease in the community.

The majority of the statistics in this contribution are derived from routine statistical systems; obviously considerable care has to be given to the interpretation of the available statistics, bearing in mind the validity of the data and the degree to which the data actually contribute to consideration of the specific aspects under consideration. My general philosophy is that the data have major problems of validity, but that with due care, there is the possibility of drawing sensible conclusions from the material. (This issue has been discussed in some detail — Alderson, 1977; 1981.)

B. Demographic aspects

The first aspect to be considered is the size of the population; England
and Wales has grown in size since censuses were first held on a regular
basis from a figure of nearly nine million in 1801 to nearly 50 million in
1981. In general, the speed of population growth has steadily declined
since these statistics first became available; by far the lowest rate of
increase was recorded at the 1981 census. When there are such major
shifts in the growth of a population, there are alterations in the age
structure. Table 1 shows the proportion of the population at various
key age-groups, including an estimate for the beginning of the next
century. It can be seen that there are changes in the percentage of the
total that can be considered 'dependent', ie children and the retired.
When grouped into the broad categories of Table 1, quite marked
changed can occur in smaller subgroups of the population, such as
those under five years of age. It is also important to remember that
only a small change in the proportion who are over 75 can have a large
impact on health and welfare requirements because the elderly are
high consumers of certain facilities.

Table 1. *Percentage age structure of England and Wales, 1901–2001.*
(1901–1981: Census reports. 2001: Population projections, Series PP2 No 10)

	1901	1921	1941	1961	1981	2001
School age or under	22.1	19.9	19.0	23.0	22.2	23.2
Working age	73.2	72.2	68.2	62.2	60.1	60.2
Pensionable age – 74	3.3	6.1	9.9	10.6	11.7	10.1
75 and over	1.4	1.7	2.9	4.3	5.8	6.5

School age 1901 — 10; 1921 — 11; 1941 — 13; 1961 — 14; 1981 and 2001 — 15.
Pensionable age 65 for males, 60 for females.

Considerable swings have occurred in the birth rate since 1945;
obviously when the number of live births per annum varies by about
30 per cent within ten years, this can be followed by changes
throughout the child age group of considerable magnitude, in terms of
facilities required for education, health, housing, and welfare.

During the present century there have been appreciable changes in
the marital structure of the country. In particular, the proportion of
women marrying has increased, and the age for marriage has altered
(Table 2). There was also a relative deficit of husbands as a result of
the first world war. The proportion of women who were widowed in
their sixties fell, because of the increased proportion that were entering

Table 2. *Percentage of women in various age groups by marital status, England and Wales, 1911–1980. (1921–71: Census reports. 1980: unpublished population estimates.)*

Year	25-29		50-54			75 +		
	Single	Married	Single	Married	Widowed	Single	Married	Widowed
1911	43.4	55.8	15.0	68.5	16.5	12.1	16.1	71.8
1921	41.0	56.8	15.9	70.0	14.0	13.2	17.1	69.6
1931	40.6	58.7	15.9	70.7	13.2	14.7	17.5	67.8
1941	28.1	71.2	16.1	69.8	14.2	16.8	16.8	66.3
1951	21.7	77.0	15.0	73.7	10.4	16.5	20.2	63.3
1961	15.7	83.5	12.2	77.8	8.4	16.0	19.1	64.8
1971	13.3	84.7	8.3	81.5	8.0	15.4	18.8	65.4
1980	16.9	78.7	6.6	81.7	7.1	14.0	19.7	65.5

this age married; however, at older age groups, the proportion of women widowed has increased, due to the relative disparity of the mortality rates in the two sexes.

The fertility of the population is best examined by use of cohort rates, following members of different cohorts through their reproductive lives. The rates may be prepared for birth or marriage cohorts, and examined by advancing age or advancing duration of marriage. Where family planning is widespread, cohort fertility is more likely to reveal underlying trends than period fertility. The influence of age at marriage on fertility can be eliminated in the marriage cohorts. Very few married couples today continue child-bearing beyond the tenth year of marriage; over 90 per cent of legitimate births occur within that time. Table 3 gives an indication of the main changes in recent years; those marrying between 1956 and 1960 achieved higher figures than earlier cohorts, but those marrying after 1960 show an appreciable fall in fertility (OPCS, 1977).

Table 3. *Average number of children born live in first marriage by duration of marriage. From Demographic review (OPCS, 1977)*

Period of first marriage	All women married for		
	2 years	5 years	10 years
1936–40	0.51	1.00	1.64
1941–45	0.52	1.14	1.74
1946–50	0.64	1.24	1.82
1951–55	0.58	1.23	1.92
1956–60	0.63	1.39	2.09
1961–65	0.69	1.45	2.05
1966–70	0.61	1.31	
1971–74	0.47		

There are variations in the age, sex and social class structure of the different regions. Table 4 shows the percentage of the population in the different standard regions in England and Wales who are in Social Class IV and V; they have been ranged in descending order, with the North West having the greatest proportion, and the South East having the least. This is only one of the many differences in the structure and characteristics of these regions.

The census of 1981 has already shown that the rate of migration into and out of the different regions varies considerably; between 1961 and

Table 4. *Percentage of persons in social class IV and V in different regions in England and Wales, 1971. (Census reports, 1971)*

Standard regions	% in IV plus V
North West	28.2
Yorkshire and Humberside	27.9
West Midlands	27.6
North	27.5
East Anglia	27.4
Wales	26.4
East Midlands	25.7
South West	23.9
South East	22.6

1971 none of the regions showed a decrease in population, but in 1971–81, five of the 'regions' in Great Britain showed a decrease. This was not as great as the changes that occurred in the central parts of the regions, with metropolitan counties from all eight conurbations in Great Britain showing a decrease in size, particularly London and Central Clydeside. Great Britain can be classified into Standard Metropolitan Labour Areas (SMLA), with labour cores made up of entire local authorities with a density of at least 12.5 workers per hectare, and surrounding metropolitan rings from which at least 15 per cent of its workers travel to the associated urban core. Outside this SMLA is a more loosely associated outer metropolitan commuter ring, the remainder of the country being considered outside the 'urban system'. The dominant trend since 1957 has been of accelerating decentralisation, with urban cores losing population to adjacent commuter hinterlands, and of spread into the outer metropolitan rings (OPCS, 1977).

Reference has already been made to the distribution of social class in the different regions. It would be of value if data on the trends of social class distribution in the country over time could be examined. However, changes have been made to the classification of social class used for successive censuses, either because of changes of the relative standing in the community of different categories of worker or as an attempt to purge the classification of weakness encountered in its use. This has been discussed in the decennial supplement on occupational mortality (OPCS, 1978a). There have been increases in the proportion of men in Social Classes I and II, and decreases in Social Class V;

Social Class III shows a confounding with age, with decreasing proportions in this class with advancing age.

The suitability of 'social class' for studying population subgroups warrants consideration. Occupation was used in the nineteenth century to probe the 'health' of various segments of the population in this country (Registrar General, 1855); this activity was extended by Stevenson (1919), who divided the population into eight social groups in studying infant mortality. This use of 'social class' derived from occupation has continued up to the present time, but has been subject to considerable controversy over its basis and application (see DHSS, 1980 for review of this issue). There have been a number of developments recently which indicate that other factors might be used to identify subgroups of the population with varying health patterns; the desiderata are that the items required for classifying individuals are readily obtained, that the basic information is reliable, that it distributes the population into subgroups of appreciable or equal size, that the groups genuinely discriminate risk of disease, and there is preferably a theoretical basis to the use of the system. Using classifying information for the 1971 census, and relating this to subsequent mortality in a cohort study of 1 per cent of the population, Fox & Goldblatt (1982) have indicated the discrimination from (a) housing tenure for households, and (b) possession of a car. These appeared to be independent associates of risk of mortality and warrant further exploration. Other work has suggested that individuals may be categorised by their address into families or clusters that were derived from a multivariate analysis of socio-economic information collected in the 1971 census; the suitability of this approach in relating the classification to subsequent indices of morbidity or mortality has yet to be demonstrated (work in progress, OPCS).

There are major differences in the growth rate of populations in different parts of the world, but it is impossible to do more than acknowledge this here. Table 5 indicates the range for a sample of countries. Though the annual percentage differences do not seem very large, it must be remembered that after 30 years the following increases in population will have occurred: 1 per cent annual increase implies growth to 135 per cent in 30 years; 2 per cent to 181 per cent; 3 per cent to 242 per cent; 4 per cent to 324 per cent. For some of the developed, and many of the developing countries, there are no data available to permit examination of these issues. For example, some countries do not have a regular census, nor statistics that permit classification of their populations by such aspects as social class or region of residence.

Table 5. *Percentage rate of increase in populations in various countries, 1975–79. (From Demographic Year Book 1979 Table 3; United Nations, New York, 1980)*

Country	%	Country	%
Africa		Asia	
Ivory Coast	4.2	China	1.4
Nigeria	3.2	India	2.8
North America		Europe	
Canada	1.1	Scotland	-0.2
Jamaica	1.4	Spain	1.1
South America		USSR	0.9
Chile	1.6		
Peru	2.8		

C. Environment

Before getting enmeshed in consideration of the various aspects of the environment that are thought to be related to the risk of disease, it is important to recollect a salutary lesson from the between-the-wars period (1919–1939) in Britain. There was then great hope that by providing modern housing people's lives might be improved. The opportunity was taken to assess this when moving families to new council estates in Stockton-on-Tees (McGonigle, 1933). The mortality of the county borough as a whole, and of a part of the area being rehoused, was used as a control when the first families were moved. Much to the surprise of the health department concerned, the mortality in those moving was increased, whilst that in control localities decreased over the same period. Though the control families were not randomly allocated, there was no reason to doubt their comparability. The main reason adduced for this rather depressing result was that the move to new housing involved additional expenditure, thus leaving inadequate money for essentials. The moral, not to be pushed too far but worthy of consideration, is that some preventive campaigns may not always have the result required or expected and that the ideal solutions to some of our health and welfare problems may not be the most obvious ones. As far as the following material is concerned, any statistical association between an environmental factor and a disease does not imply cause and effect, and more

Table 6. *Percentage of households without exclusive use of various facilities, England and Wales, 1951–1981. (Census reports 1951–1981)*

	Cold water %	Hot water %	Bath %	WC %
1951	12	. .	38	14
1961	4	24	27	13
1971	. .	8	12	5
1981	. .	. .	3	. .

Table 7. *Percentage of households living at varying density levels in England and Wales, 1921–1981. (Census housing reports 1921–1981)*

Year	>2.0 %	>1.5 %	>1.0 %
1921	5.7	16.3	34.0
1931	3.9	11.5	26.1
1951	1.2	5.1	16.0
1961	. .	2.8	10.3
1971	. .	1.4	5.9
1981	. .	. .	3.4

important, removing the influence of the factor in question may not result in an improvement in health.

Considering the housing of this country first, the censuses since 1951 have recorded the sharing or lack of various facilities, such as piped water, cooking stoves, kitchen sinks, water closets, fixed baths, or hot water. Though the data have not been published in a standard way from one census to the next, there have been major changes in the provision of such facilities. The proportion of households lacking exclusive use of these facilities is given in Table 6. Related to this is the degree to which households may be considered to be overcrowded. The number of persons per household, and the number of rooms available for the household have been recorded since before the turn of the century, and Table 7 presents trends in the more recent statistics. (It must be borne in mind that the definitions of some of the terms may have altered during this period, and the data have not always been published in a way that identical statistical categories may be retrieved). Perhaps of greater relevance to nutrition is the information

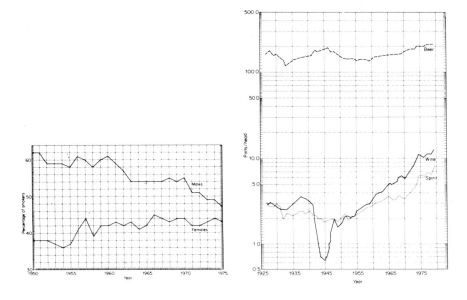

Fig. 1. *Percentage of men and women aged 16 and over, smoking, United Kingdom, 1950–1975. (Alderson, 1982)*

Fig. 2. *Beer, wine and spirit consumption per head of population, United Kingdom, 1927–1979. (Alderson, 1982)*

about possession of a refrigerator, which has been recorded in the General Household Survey since 1972 (see OPCS, 1982).

Turning now to certain facets of behaviour, and briefly considering smoking, drinking and diet, there are a wealth of statistics published on these topics and only limited comment will be made (see Alderson, 1982 for a review on this topic). Over the past 40 years there have been appreciable changes in the smoking habits of the public. The percentage of males smoking has steadily decreased over the past 25 years; though the number of cigarettes smoked has increased, this has been more than offset by a reduction in their tar content. The trends for women have been quite different, with a tendency to increase, especially in the younger segments of the population. There are differences in the social class distribution of smoking and trends in smoking; independently, there are changes in the proportion smoking in different regions of the UK. The same may be said for alcohol consumption, except that this is a more complex subject involving three main types of alcoholic beverage. Limited data are presented

on this in Figs 1 and 2. The fairly complex changes that have occurred
in the dietary patterns of this country have recently been described
(Turner & Gray, 1982). In summary, it may be noted that there have
been appreciable changes in the habits of this country, as far as food/
drink/cigarette consumption is concerned; these changes may be
different in the regions of the country or in different segments of the
populations (ie by sex, age, or social class).

Turning now to the issues related to occupation, a simple issue is the
proportion of women who have worked at different times in this
century. Table 8 shows that the proportion has gradually increased
since 1901, irrespective of any confounding changes in the age
structure of the population within the conventional age span at which
women have worked. It must be borne in mind that this table simplifies
a complex set of changes that have occurred; there have been major
changes in the range of jobs that were available — with an appreciable
proportion being in service industries at the beginning of the century,
and an increasing number in clerical and assembly work in more
recent times. There have been major changes in the occupations
followed by men this century, with a steady decrease in the proportion
involved in agriculture, mining and quarrying, textiles, and
woodworking; over the same period there has been an appreciable rise
in the proportion involved in desk-bound jobs — professional, administrative, and clerical. This change in the profile of jobs has been
accompanied by an alteration in the number of hours usually worked,
with a steady decrease since before 1939 for both men and women
(from 47.7 to 43.2 for men, and 43.5 to 37.5 hours for women). Thus
there have been two quite different changes — the proportion of men
involved in heavy physical labour has decreased and the amount of
time available for leisure has increased. There have also been changes
in the way in which leisure is spent — the cinema has declined
markedly in popularity, watching television has become a major
consumer of time, and the proportion of men spending time at
spectator sport has varied, with reduction in attending football
matches being partly offset by attendance at other sport (see Social
Trends 1982, 1981). With a relative increase in the earnings of manual
workers, the way holidays are spent has altered; there has been an
increase in time spent away from home, rather than on day trips, and
with an appreciable increase in the amount of foreign travel.

Turning briefly to the direct or indirect effect of industrial change in
Britain on the environment, there has been a major increase in the
production of organic chemicals — an increase of about 330 per cent in
the period 1963–1979. Using a specific example that is at least

Table 8. *Percentage of women employed for Census Years 1901-71 England and Wales*

Year	Age	% Employed women
1901	10 + over	24.8
1911	10 + over	25.9
1921	12 + over	25.6
1931	14 + over	26.9
1951	15 + over	27.6
1961	15 + over	28.9
1971	15 + over	31.6

indirectly related to the topic of nutrition, the production of fertilizer has increased to a modest extent in this country: from 1713 thousand tonnes in 1949 to 2797 thousand tonnes in 1979.

These points are made in order to quantify the various changes that have occurred in the home and general environment and not to assert that the changes are automatically associated with any change in the general risk to health.

D. Health of the population

There are very limited statistics on the health of the population; because of this, I have made use of some measureable events that are only indirectly suitable as indices of health. A traditional one is the expectation of life — this might be rationalised by remembering that one has at least to be alive in order to be healthy. Figure 3 shows the increase of expectation of life that has occurred in England & Wales during the period 1841-1975. The Figure relates to individuals who have reached their fifteenth birthday, whose expectation is less than that for a newborn child, despite the relatively high mortality that afflicts the newborn. The Figure suggests that the change has been fairly gradual during the entire period; it is perhaps salutary to note that there has not been a major change with the advent of modern medicine, but that there were improvements before the advent of antibiotics and the advances in hospital care that have been achieved in the past thirty years. Another point to note is the steady increment in life expectancy of women over that of men; some of the reasons for

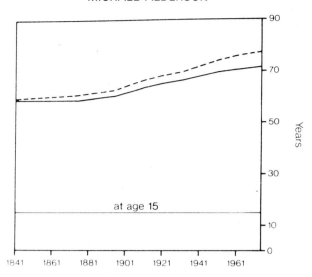

Fig. 3. *Expectation of age at death for those reaching age 15, England and Wales, 1841–1975. Males:* ———, *females:* -------. *OPCS (1978b).*

this will be discussed in a later section. If one examines the trend in life expectancy for an older age-group, such as those who have achieved the age of 45, the relative increase is not so great. (It is worth noting that Benjamin (In press) has examined cohort life tables for Britain, disagreeing with the view that there is a finite limit to the time span of an individual's life; he suggested that with improvement in the environment and in medical care there will be an increasing proportion of individuals surviving to advanced ages.) Comparable data may be examined for other countries in the world, provided that registration of vital statistics exists; there is very little difference in the expectation for most of the developed countries (in fact the difference in expectation of life between males and females in England and Wales is greater than the difference between males in England and Wales and males in other developed countries). However, there is a lack of adequate information for many of the developing countries — some of them would have figures very different from countries in Western Europe.

Another simple way of looking at the health of the community is to examine the trends in mortality from all causes; this may be examined as a crude rate, or preferably as an age-standardised rate, adjusted for the variation in the age distribution of the population (otherwise a region or country with a higher proportion of elderly would appear to

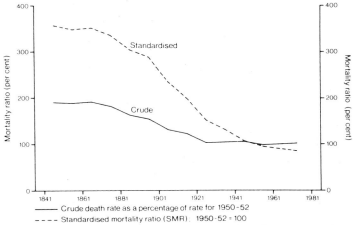

Fig. 4. *Trends in mortality, persons, England and Wales, 1841–1975. OPCS (1978b).*

have a high mortality rate). Figure 4 shows that in England and Wales there has been a decrease in crude mortality during the period 1841–1975. When the ageing effect of the population is taken into account, the standardised rate shows an even more marked decline. However, this change has not been even throughout the community; if age-specific rates are examined for males and females quite marked differences appear. The decrease has been greatest for the youngest age-groups, especially those aged 0–4, 5–9, and 10–14 years; in the oldest age groups, there has been very little improvement. There are also easily detected changes in the shape of the curves for males compared to females; the rates for women have improved to a greater extent, both for adolescents and the very elderly. (This material has been presented in Trends in Mortality, OPCS 1978b).

A more subtle index of the health of a community is the infant mortality rate, or its components (still births, deaths in the first week of life, the first month of life, or the remainder of the first year of life). Figure 5 shows the trend in some of these statistics for England and Wales since the 1930s (stillbirths were only registered from 1927, hence the absence of earlier data). Figure 5 shows an appreciable decrease in the mortality rates of the infants born over the past 50 years. However, it must be remembered that there are variations in the risk of such deaths in different segments of the community; the rates are higher in some parts of the country than others (ie high in the North and West), whilst there is appreciable difference in the rates for the different social classes (see Adelstein *et al.*, 1980 for a discussion of this topic). Recent studies have indicated complex inter-relationships, for example deaths of infants aged 1-11 months are more common where mothers (a) are 20 years old, (b) have had at least three previous pregnancies. Young mothers having their fourth child form a very high-risk group (Adelstein *et al.*, 1982).

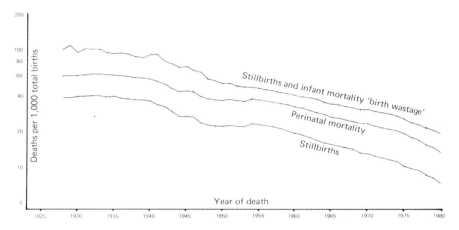

Fig. 5. *Stillbirths, perinatal mortality, and stillbirths and infant mortality per thousand total births, England and Wales, 1928-1980. Based on GRO, OPCS annual mortality statistics.*

Compared with the expectation of life, there are appreciable international differences in infant mortality, even in Europe — there are major differences between Greece or Spain and Scandinavian countries. The range is very great between one part of the world and another, even though data are not routinely available for many developing countries.

Recently the General Household Survey, which is a major survey carried out annually by the Social Survey Division of the Office of Population Censuses and Surveys using a sample throughout Great Britain, has introduced a question asking respondents to state whether they consider their health 'Good', 'Fairly good', or 'Not good' (OPCS, 1979). This will now provide some data on the view of the population about their general state of health. Table 9 sets out some of the results obtained in 1979. It can be seen that the proportion thinking their health was 'Not good' increased with advancing age; for persons over the age of 65, a higher proportion of women than men gave this answer (an interesting contrast with the better mortality experience of women

Table 9. *Percentage of persons reporting various levels of health in preceding year, Great Britain, 1979 From General Household Survey, 1980 (OPCS 1982)*

Age	Good		Fairly good		Not good	
	M	F	M	F	M	F
16–	77	69	19	24	4	7
45–	57	52	29	33	14	15
65–	45	39	34	36	22	25
75+	38	28	36	38	25	34

compared with men). This view of the 'health' is the only such measure that we have.

The next section turns to the consideration of statistics about disease in the community (obtained predominantly from contact with the health service); it is important to remember that some people do not contact their doctor, even though suffering from readily identifiable disease (see Alderson & Dowie, 1979 for a review of this topic). The picture of the health of the community is thus rather incomplete and lacks any objective measure of mental and physical health of the community.

E. Illness in the community

This section turns to some of the available statistics on illness in the community, dealing first with further data from the General Household Survey and then contact with the general practitioners; the main difference in the statistics collected from general practice is that the diagnoses are provided from the doctors' records whilst no diagnostic information is now collected in the General Household Survey. Hospital discharge records provide another source of information which relates to an important component of 'disease in the community' or treatment in hospital. Finally, brief consideration of the patterns of mortality in England and Wales can draw upon statistics from by far the longest time series of data — some material is available from the early part of the nineteenth century — though diagnostic and other aspects of validity have to be very carefully considered when examining long-term trends.

The General Household Survey records several different items within the health section; statistics on restricted activity and longstanding illness are shown in Table 10. Obviously the full reports should be consulted for detail on the method of obtaining this material. The data show that there is a marked increase in reported illness with advancing age and in the older age-groups the females report a higher prevalence of disability. There is also a much higher prevalence of longstanding disability than restricted activity in the older age-groups.

Table 10. *Percentage of persons reporting illness in Great Britain, 1979. (General Household Survey, 1982)*

Age	Lond-standing illness		Restricted activity	
	M	F	M	F
0–	8	6	12	10
5–	14	10	11	11
15–	21	20	10	13
45–	39	38	14	14
65–	50	52	12	16
75+	56	64	27	22

The statistics from the General Practice Studies co-ordinated by the Royal College of General Practitioners, the Department of Health and Social Security and the Office of Population Censuses and Surveys provide an extensive set of statistics and it is only possible to select a very minor component. Table 11 compares the contact rate of patients with their general practitioners with the discharge rate from acute hospitals (ie excluding psychiatric and maternity units) for the same selected conditions. Five common disorders affecting men and women have been chosen, in order to show the major differences in the levels of contact with these two branches of the health service. For both sexes there is approximately a ten-fold difference in the statistics; the major exception is intracranial injuries, where obviously the nature of this is likely to require hospital care. Even for malignant disease of the lung, though not ten-fold, there are considerably more contacts with the general practitioner than admissions to hospital. It is also worth noting that there is an appreciable difference in the rates for different diseases; rather different diseases also appear in the table for either sex and this is a genuine reflection of the difference in the patterns of morbidity in the two sexes.

Turning now to consideration of patterns of mortality, the first issue

Table 11. *Discharge'rates per 1000 from NHS hospitals in 1978 and contact rates in general practice 1972, England and Wales. From Hospital in-patient enquiry, 1978 (DHSS, 1982); Morbidity statistics from general practice, 1971–2 (RCPG/OPCS/DHSS, 1979)*

Condition	Hospital discharge	GP contact
Males aged 45–64:		
Myocardial infarction	5.6	83.9
Abdominal pain	1.2	17.3
Hernia	5.2	24.5
Lung cancer	3.0	13.0
Intracranial injury	1.3	1.9
Females aged 45–64:		
Breast cancer	3.1	20.4
Abdominal pain	1.4	26.6
Cerebrovascular disease	1.7	18.9
Arthritis and spondylitis	2.5	31.3
Cholelithiasis and cholecysitis	2.4	15.7

is the relative numbers of deaths at different ages and the relative patterns of disease by cause in the different age groups. This aspect involves a complex set of statistics and some of the material is thus presented in a highly condensed form. Numerically, there are relatively few deaths in the young, but an appreciable increase in the age group 35–54 years; by this age the causes of death begin to stabilise, and are comparable with further advance in age — though there are some notable differences between the sexes. In both males and females there are more deaths in the age group 55–74 years than in the over 75s; this is a reflection of the much larger number of the population below the age of 75, though the age-specific rates are higher with advancing age. Table 12 sets out the main statistics of mortality by cause and age; it is interesting to note how relatively few conditions account for the majority of deaths, with a large number of other conditions causing a few additional deaths.

There is variation in the force of mortality affecting the different social classes — both for all causes and specific causes. One aspect of this issue has been explored by Fox & Goldblatt (1982), using classifying information from the 1971 census and relating this to subsequent mortality in a cohort study of 1 per cent of the population of England and Wales. They showed appreciable variation in mortality rate

Table 12. *Five main causes of death at different ages (and percentage of all cause deaths) England and Wales, 1980. Criteria for entry into the table was the 'cause' did not extend over more than ten ICD 3-digit rubrics (thus giving a minimum cause list of 99 and a maximum of 999 causes considered for entry). (OPCS 1982 — Unpublished data.)*

Rank	All ages				1-14				15-44			
	Males	%	Females	%	Males	%	Females	%	Males	%	Females	%
1	Ischaemic heart disease	22	Ischaemic heart disease	31	Motor vehicle traffic accidents	17	Motor vehicle traffic accidents	12	Motor vehicle traffic accidents	19	MN of: Bone connective tissue, skin and breast	14
2	MN of Respiratory and intra-thoracic organs	15	Cerebrovascular disease	10	MN of: Lymphatic and haematopoietic tissue	8	MN of: Lymphatic and haematopoietic tissue	8	Ischaemic heart disease	15	Motor vehicle traffic accidents	8
3	Cerebrovascular disease	11	Pneumonia and influenza	9	Accident caused by by submersion, suffocation and foreign bodies	7	Pneumonia and influenza	7	Suicide	10	Suicide	7
4	Pneumonia and influenza	7	MN of: Digestive organs and peritoneum	8	Pneumonia and influenza	6	Bulbus cordis anomalies	6	MN of: Lymphatic and haematopoietic tissue	4	Cerebrovascular disease	6
5	MN of: Digestive organs and peritoneum	5	MN of: Bone, connective tissue, skin and breast	7	Bulbus cordis anomalies	4	MN of: Brain	4	MN of: Digestive organs and peritoneum	4	MN of: Digestive organs and peritoneum	5
Remainder		40		35		58		64		48		60
All causes of death	291869	100	289516	100	1731	100	1240	100	12271	100	6995	100

Table 12 (continued)

Rank	45–64				65–84				75 +			
	Males	%	Females	%	Males	%	Females	%	Males	%	Females	%
1	Ischaemic heart disease	40	Ischaemic heart disease	18	Ischaemic heart disease	31	Ischaemic heart disease	26	Ischaemic heart disease	22	Pneumonia and influenza	20
2	MN of: Respiratory and intra-thoracic organs	13	MN of: Bone, connective tissue, skin and breast	13	Cerebrovascular disease	13	Cerebrovascular disease	16	Pneumonia and influenza	16	Ischaemic heart disease	˙19
3	MN of: Digestive organs and peritoneum	9	MN of: Digestive organs and peritoneum	9	MN of: Respiratory and intra-thoratic organs	10	Pneumonia and influenza	10	Cerebrovascular disease	13	Cerebrovascular disease	18
4	Cerebrovascular disease	8	Cerebrovascular disease	6	Pneumonia and influenza	8	MN of: Digestive organs and peritoneum	8	Chronic obstructive pulmonary disease	7	Disease of arteries, arterioles/capillaries	5
5	Chronic obstructive pulmonary disease	8	MN of: Respiratory and intra-thoracic organs	4	Chronic obstructive pulmonary disease	7	MN of: Bone, connective tissue, skin and breast	7	MN of: Digestive organs and peritoneum	4	Heart failure	4
Remainder		44		28		33		37		35		34
All causes of death	65746	100	38614	100	179488	100	166815	100	28162	100	72424	100

(adjusted for age distribution: Standard Mortality Ratio = SMR) in 1971-75 in those males aged 15-64 in 1971 who were, at census recorded as: in employment (SMR 86); off work, sick (SMR 323); seeking work (SMR 130); retired (SMR 153); permanently sick (SMR 392); student (SMR 83); inactive for other reasons (SMR 105). This is a warning of the danger of pooling data for these different subgroups.

Of greater interest for this presentation are the time trends of some of these conditions and the variation that occurs in different parts of the country. The great decrease in overall mortality this century has already been discussed in the previous section; Figs 6 and 7 show how the trends have run for seven main categories of disease. The commonest cause of death in males is cardiovascular disease; it is now clearly so, but appears to have achieved this position chiefly due to the decrease in mortality from other causes. The second commonest cause is now malignant neoplasms, which have increased in absolute and relative terms. At the same time there have been some appreciable decreases — particularly for infectious diseases — but also for respiratory, alimentary, and genito-urinary disease. Women present a

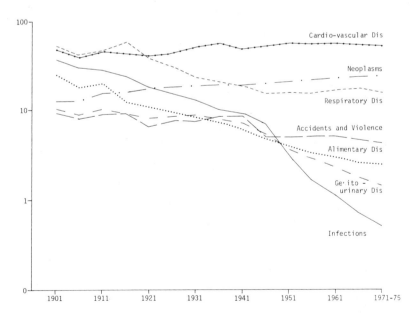

Fig. 6. *Age-adjusted trends in mortality rates, for various causes for males, England and Wales 1901-1975. Based on Alderson (1981).*

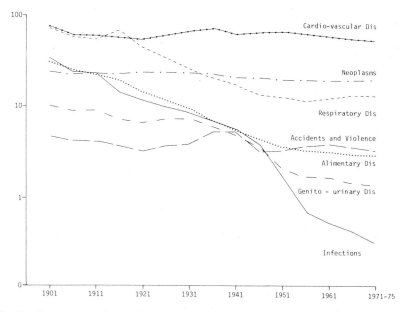

Fig. 7. *Age-adjusted trends in mortality rates, for various causes for females, England and Wales 1901–1975. Based on Alderson (1981).*

similar picture; the one main exception that may be noted is the slight decrease in malignant diseases that has occurred — this is due to the much more rapid rise that occurred in the earlier part of this century in lung cancer in males, but not in females. It must be acknowledged that by using very broad conditions such as appear in Figs 6 and 7 other marked differences in specific causes of death can be lost.

In order to consider the geographical distribution of disease, it is important to note that there are confounding factors that may distort the simple comparison of one area of England and Wales with another. If one location has a population made up of a very different age-distribution to that for the whole country, one might expect variation of mortality that is quite unrelated to any direct geographical effect (this principle applies to other comparisons that are made throughout this presentation — thus an industry may have a different population age structure which needs to be taken into account before making comparisons). It has already been pointed out that there is variation in the social class mortality, with high mortality for all causes in Social Class V. As the proportion of persons in the different classes varies throughout the country, it is useful to examine the regional variation

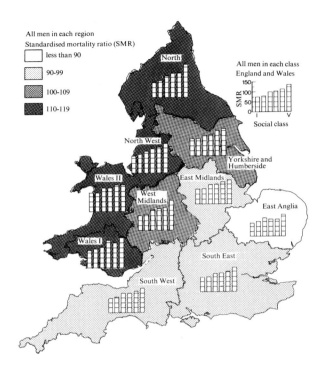

Fig. 8. *All cause standardised mortality ratios for males, 15–64, by social class and region, England and Wales 1970–1972. From Fox (1977).*

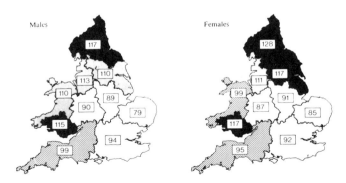

Fig. 9. *Standardised mortality ratios for acute myocardial infarction in males and females, England and Wales, 1969–1973. OPCS (1981b).*

in mortality within the social classes; Figure 8 shows how the gradient remains in the different regions, but the overall level of mortality varies from one region to another.

Bearing the above point in mind, the areal variation in mortality can be examined for various diseases. As an example, Fig. 9 shows data for deaths from acute myocardial infarction for males and females in England and Wales in 1969-73. Analyses were published for 100 different causes, with age adjusted rates down to the level of country boroughs (OPCS, 1981*b*).

References

Adelstein, A. M. *et al.* (1980): *Perinatal and Infant Mortality: Social and Biological Factors, 1975-1977.* Studies on Medical and Population Subjects, No. 41. London: HMSO.

Adelstein, A. M. *et al.* (1981): *Studies in Infant Deaths.* Studies on Medical and Population Subjects, No. 45. London: HMSO.

Alderson, M. R. (1977): *An Introduction to Epidemiology.* London: Macmillan.

Alderson, M. R. (1981): *International Mortality Statistics.* London: Macmillan.

Alderson, M. R. (editor) (1982): *The Prevention of Cancer.* London: Edward Arnold.

Alderson, M. R. & Dowie, R. (1979): *Health Surveys and Related Studies.* Oxford: Pergamon.

Benjamin, B. (In press): The Span of Life. *Journal of Institute of Actuaries.*

Department of Health and Social Security (1980): *Inequalities in Health: a Report of a Research Working Party.* London: DHSS.

Department of Health and Social Security, Office of Population Censuses and Surveys, Welsh Office (1981): *Hospital In-Patient Enquiry 1978.* London: HMSO.

Fox, A. J. (1977): Occupational mortality. *Population Trends* 9, 8-15. London: HMSO.

Fox, A. J. & Goldblatt, P. O. (1982): *Longitudinal Study: Socio-Economic Mortality Differentials, 1971-75 England and Wales.* London: HMSO.

McGonigle, G. C. M. (1933): Poverty, nutrition, and the public health. *Proceedings of the Royal Society of Medicine* 26, 677-687.

Office of Population Censuses and Surveys (1977): *Demographic Review.* London: OPCS.

Office of Population Censuses and Surveys (1978*a*): *Occupational Mortality: Decennial Supplement England and Wales, 1970-72.* London: HMSO.

Office of Population Censuses and Surveys (1978*b*): *Trends in Mortality, DH1 No. 3.* London: HMSO.

Office of Population Censuses and Surveys (1979): *General Household Survey 1977*. London: HMSO.

Office of Population Censuses and Surveys (1981*a*): *General Household Survey 1979*. London: HMSO.

Office of Population Censuses and Surveys (1981*b*): *Area Mortality 1969–73, DS No. 4*. London: HMSO.

Office of Population Censuses and Surveys (1982): *General Household Survey 1980*. London: HMSO.

Registrar General (1855): *14th Annual Report of the Registrar General of Births, Deaths and Marriages in England*. London: HMSO.

Royal College of General Practitioners, Office of Population Censuses and Surveys, Department of Health and Social Security (1979): *Morbidity Statistics from General Practice 1971–72. Second National Study*. Studies on Medical and Population Subjects, No. 36. London: HMSO.

Stevenson, T. A. C. (1919): *Supplement to the 75th annual report of the Registrar General for England and Wales, Part IV: Mortality of men in Certain Occupations 1910–12*. London: HMSO.

Social trends 1982 (1981): London: Central Statistical Office, HMSO.

Turner, M. R. & Gray, J. R. (1982): *Implementation of Dietary Guidelines*. London: British Nutrition Foundation.

2

Social class, poverty and nutrition

MILDRED BLAXTER

A. Introduction

Dr Alderson's paper in this volume has demonstrated that, despite the changing socio-economic profile of the British population and the changing patterns of disease and mortality, occupational class (as defined by the Registrar General) is still an important variable in the analysis of health and sickness. Here I shall attempt to consider why this should be so — what is the real meaning of 'social class' in this context? What is its relationship to poverty, and what evidence is there that poverty is associated with poor nutrition in contemporary Britain? Are we really talking of a level of resources so low that it prevents the purchasing of adequate nourishment?

It is necessary, first, briefly to distinguish the concepts involved in the definition and measurement of poverty. The first is *absolute poverty*, which was the concept used by Seerbohm Rowntree in 1899 in York, in the first detailed poverty study (Rowntree, 1901). Rowntree defined primary poverty as 'total earnings which are insufficient to obtain the minimum necessaries for the maintenance of merely physical efficiency', and the poverty line was set at 17 shillings and 8 pence a week, plus rent, for a couple and three children, 12 shillings and 9 pence of which was for food. A family in primary poverty so defined, Rowntree noted,

> '. . . must never spend a penny on railway fare or omnibus. . . . They must never purchase a halfpenny newspaper or spend a penny to buy a ticket for a popular concert. . . . The children must have no pocket money for dolls, marbles or sweets. . . . The father must smoke no tobacco and drink no beer'.

The aim of this survey, and of the 1936 survey (Rowntree, 1937) which defined subsistence only slightly less stringently, was to show irrefutably that poverty did exist. Ironically, however, this restrictive definition became the basis upon which the original welfare state was erected (Kincaid, 1975). Obviously, an 'absolute' concept of poverty raises problems. Requirements for food, at least, may be held to be based on scientific standards. But the nutritional estimates which Beveridge used in his calculation of 'minimum needs' (Beveridge, 1942) were broad averages, not varied by age or work or family composition, and the scales made assumptions about consuming behaviour which were unrealistic. Subsistence budgets ensure minimum living standards only if families spend their money in the exact manner specified, and since families vary, some will by definition be below subsistence. For items other than food, Beveridge's standards were derived from the expenditure of working-class households in the 1937 Family Budget Survey, producing a circular definition: income obviously determines choice, but choice is used to measure need.

A second concept for the measurement of poverty is a *relative* one. Thus one may take account of the general historical rise in the standard of living, acknowledging that what is held to be an acceptable subsistence level will change over time. If one takes, at adjusted value, the absolute poverty line in 1953 as standard, for instance, by 1973 the extent of poverty had contracted to only one-tenth of the proportion of the population 20 years before (Fiegehen *et al.*, 1977) (though it must be noted that this still means that there was a small proportion which had an income below the minimum of 20 years previously).

To measure the extent of relative poverty one may select, arbitrarily, the lowest 5 or 10 per cent — or any other percentage — of the population and define these as the relatively poor. Or one may relate incomes to the median for the society, and declare that the poor are those who have a given fraction, say half of median income.

In practice, the poverty line operated by the State in Britain is an absolute one, with some admixture of relative elements. The Supplementary Benefit level expresses, at any one time, the current national concept of a minimum tolerable level. The long-term rate is set, in a relative fashion, at about one half of the national average. Because of the issue already mentioned about variability in needs and behaviour, it is common, when using Supplementary Benefit (SB) scales to estimate the numbers in poverty, to add an arbitrary 20 or 40 per cent, and talk of '<120 per cent SB'. Indeed, practice confirms this, since the actual amounts paid contain disregards and special additional payments. But another problem arises because of the development, since 1966, of two scale rates. Originally, the higher long-term rate was intended to cover the small exceptional needs of the sick and elderly, but the two rates have now diverged by 27 per cent.

Since there cannot be two absolute levels, this means either that the State has decided to raise some people 27 per cent above subsistence, or that the basic rate is in fact inadequate. The evidence suggests the latter. The Supplementary Benefit Commission itself had for some years argued that the basic scales are too low (Donnison, 1981), and nutritional analyses have suggested that the allowance for children is inadequate to cover their food needs, even with the most 'efficient' purchasing pattern (Walker & Church, 1978).

So, in counting the number of households in poverty in Britain, one may use either the basic rate, the long-term rate, or the long-term rate adjusted for children (since it applies to the needs of adults only). As Table 1 shows, very different estimates will be obtained.

Table 1. *Poverty by Supplementary Benefit (SB) standards, 1975. From Berthoud* et al. *(1981)*

Households below:	Number ('000)
Basic SB level	880
Long-term SB level	2560
Long-term level adjusted for children	2890

It may be asked: why, if this is the State's minimum subsistence rate, are there *any* households below it? The answer is, of course, that some are not eligible, and some do not apply. Table 2 shows the proportions of households in Britain above and below the minimum poverty line, and the proportions lifted above it by the receipt of benefits or left below it because they are not receiving benefits. Other studies

Table 2. *Poverty and receipt of social security benefits, 1971. From Fiegehen* et al. *(1977)*

	%	
	Receiving benefits	Not receiving benefits
Households with income:		
Below SB poverty line	2.7	4.4
Above SB poverty line	9.9	83.0

SB = Supplementary Benefit.

estimating entitlement to benefits have found higher proportions who have not taken them up.

There is, however, a third concept of poverty, sometimes called the *behaviouristic*, which emphasises its relative nature and goes beyond income. Townsend defines it thus:

> Individuals, families and groups in the population can be said to be in poverty when they lack the resources to obtain the types of diet, participate in the activities, and have the living conditions which are necessary, or at least widely encouraged or approved, in the societies to which they belong (Townsend, 1979).

Similarly, the Report to Parliament of the Supplementary Benefits Commission in 1978 presented the issue squarely:

> To keep out of poverty people must have an income which enables them to participate in the life of the community.

Poverty is thus defined as a relatively low score on a broadly defined dimension, an overall living standard. In his *Poverty Survey*, Townsend (1979) operationalised this by measuring the level of income (for different population groups) below which people were unable to participate in what were judged to be the normal conventions of their society. He found that average participation varied little between the broad range of income groups, but fell off rapidly below a certain income level. This cut-off point between normal and reduced participation lay at about 138 per cent of basic Supplementary Benefit rates, and this he called the 'deprivation standard' of income.

B. The extent and distribution of poverty

These three concepts of poverty produce different estimates of its extent, as shown in Table 3. This is not merely academic, for differing definitions of poverty are closely associated with the social policy — including nutritional policy — designed to alleviate deprivation. An absolute standard suggests conditional welfare for the few, identifying and relieving those who fall below it. A relative view suggests an attempt, by redistributive taxation and universal benefits, to diminish inequalities. A behaviouristic view suggests that the aim should be distributional equality, not simply of income but of those resources which are not wholly controlled by the market: education, housing and health services. Welfare milk only for the most needy might be an expression of the first view, vitamin supplements for all pregnant women an expression of the second, and attempts to improve health education or to control the nutritional value of foods most commonly eaten an expression of the third.

Table 3. *Poverty by various measures, 1968–69. From Townsend (1979)*

	% of households
SB standard, in poverty	7.1
on margins	23.8
Relative standard (<50% of mean income)	9.2
on margins	29.6
Townsend's deprivation standard	22.9

SB = Supplementary Benefit.

The statistics used as examples in this paper may be based on any one of these standards, and this must be borne in mind when considering them. There are also many technical complications in the measurement of poverty which it is not possible to take into account here — the issues, for instance, of counting households or individuals, or using income or expenditure, and deciding the period over which income is to be measured. Measuring poverty on the basis of the nuclear family rather than the total household, for instance, has the effect of raising the estimated numbers by more than three-quarters (Fiegehen *et al.*, 1977). The basis of family life is that the elderly and infirm will be to some extent supported: if they are assessed on their own income, poverty will appear to rise. Also, it must be remembered that poverty is not necessarily a static condition, and many people move in and out of it at short intervals.

We may now ask, however, who are the poor, and what is the relationship of poverty to social class? One problem is that the Registrar General's definition of social class, used so successfully for very many years in exploring health relationships, is seen as less meaningful and is less frequently used for other sorts of statistics. The occupational classes used in Table 4 are only approximate to Registrar General's social classes. However, it becomes obvious that occupational class *is*, as we all know, related to income, but those in poverty are certainly not all to be placed in social classes IV and V. Using Townsend's deprivation standard, in Table 5, the gradient is steeper but the same conclusion applies.

Table 4. *Poverty by occupation.*
(General Household Survey, 1979)

	% of households with income per week	
	<£30	<£50
Head of household:		
Professional	1	2
Employers and managerial	5	13
Intermediate non-manual	5	15
Junior non-manual	14	33
Skilled manual	7	20
Semi-skilled manual, service	23	43
Unskilled manual	28	54

Table 5. *Occupation and deprivation.*
From Townsend (1979).

	% of persons below Townsend's standard
Professional	5
Managerial	6
Supervisory (high)	11
Supervisory (low)	19
Routine non-manual	27
Skilled manual	28
Partly skilled manual	30
Unskilled manual	54

Analysing by demographic variables rather than social class, it becomes obvious that the greatest *numbers* of those in poverty are to be found among the elderly, followed by couples with 1–3 children, and by single-parent families (Layard *et al.*, 1978). Looking, however, at the *proportions* of different household types which are likely to be in poverty, the old are again most likely, but amongst those below retiring age it is single parents and large families who have the greatest likelihood of being poor.

Table 6. *Estimates of populations in poverty 1975. From Layard* et al. *(1978)*

	Thousands	
Individuals in families	at or below Supplementary Benefit	100–120% Supplementary Benefit
Elderly	2190	1700
Childless couples	230	160
Couples with 1–3 children	750	1310
4 children	230	360
5 + children	220	280
Single parent families	670	340
Single men or women	300	270

Table 7. *Households with incomes below Supplementary Benefit level. From Fiegehen et al. (1977).*

All households	% in poverty
Retired males	29.0
Retired females	29.6
Retired couple	16.8
Couple, 1 child	2.5
Couple, 5 + children	13.8
Single parent, 1 child	12.7
Single parent, 3 + children	25.6

For large families, the probability is demonstrated in Table 8: 68 per cent of those with five or more children are below 140 per cent of Supplementary Benefit. For single-parent families, it is shown in Table 9 that single, divorced, or separated women with children are very likely to be in poverty. Other groups which might be singled out are the long-term unemployed or sick, the disabled, and low wage-earners with families.

Table 8. *Poverty in large families. From Layard et al. (1978).*

	% of all families with 5 + children
Family with income:	
At or below SB	20
Below 140% SB	68

SB = Supplementary Benefit.

Table 9. *Poverty in single-parent families. From Layard et al. (1978).*

	% of families with income less than 120% SB
Parent who is:	
Single woman	63
Widow	36
Separated woman	62
Divorced woman	69
Lone man	14
(All 2-parent families)	(10)

SB = Supplementary Benefit.

C. Poverty and nutrition

Are we then to conclude that poverty in Britain today is rather more a demographic phenomenon than a social class one? Is it only among these particular groups that there is likely to be deprivation which — at least in part through poor nutrition — could affect health adversely? Certainly, there is little evidence in Britain of overt nutritional deficiency which applies at the level of a whole social class, rather than applying to particular groups who are likely to be identified as belonging to lower occupational classes.

That there is evidence about particular groups such as the poor elderly (Exton-Smith, 1979; Lawson *et al.*, 1979), families of minority races (Ruck, 1979; Goel, 1979), and families in inner urban areas (Donnet & Stanfield, 1977) must be acknowledged. That nutritional evidence is lacking about others, such as the children of one-parent families, may only be because it has not been sought. The elderly are considered elsewhere in this volume, and it is children, and perhaps child-bearing women, who are the focus of the remainder of this paper.

One example of a group of children about whom evidence of nutritional deficiency is clear, is of course the children of minority races. During the 1950s the children of Asian immigrants to Britain began to present in quite large numbers with nutritional rickets, and the persistence of adolescent and later rickets and osteomalacia has been very well studied and documented in subsequent years (Benson *et al.*, 1963; Richards *et al.*, 1968; Manchester Community Health Group, 1980). In 1977 the Community Relations Commission (1977) drew attention to this and other nutritional diseases, and the topic is still a cause for concern in medical literature. Since 1979, Asian children in Glasgow have been receiving vitamin D supplementation, and it is claimed that rickets in young children has been largely suppressed, though the disease persists in post-pubertal Asians (Goel *et al.*, 1981).

Table 10. *Discharges with nutritional rickets and osteomalacia from Glasgow hospitals 1968-78. From Goel et al. (1981).*

Age (years)	numbers	
	White	Asian
0–4	25	30
5–16	2	90
17–49	0	18

It is not only dietary vitamin D deficiency, as part of the etiology of rickets, that is indicted, however. Table 11 offers some evidence from one of many surveys of the diets of immigrant children, in this case schoolgirls aged 12–17 years in Leicester (Pearson *et al.*, 1977). And, returning to Glasgow, Table 12 gives some results from a particularly careful dietary survey of children of different races (Goel, 1979). It demonstrates that each race has its own patterns, and this of course points to the fact that what we are talking about may not be a phenomenon associated with poverty or social class, but with cultural habits. But it also demonstrates something else: it can be noted that *Scots*-born children, from the same areas, suffered dietary deficiency.

Table 11. *Nutrient intake of immigrant schoolgirls in Leicester. From Pearson* et al. *(1977)*

	% with less than recommended intake
Vitamin D	99
Calcium	53
Protein	64
Energy	48
Iron	77
Vitamin B$_{12}$	81

Table 12. *Deficiencies in nutrition of infants, Glasgow. From Goel (1979)*

	% with deficient intake of:		
	Vit. D	*Calcium*	*Iron*
Scots	31	1	33
Asians	41	12	45
Africans	22	6	25
Chinese	51	11	38

Less than optimum diets, though they may not be technically deficient, have certainly been similarly recorded, especially in the infants of families in poor circumstances. Again in Glasgow, cohorts of babies who lived in areas defined as deprived were compared with a representative area; 16.7 per cent were judged to be underfed at

1 month in the deprived area, but very few in the comparison area. (It must be added that more were found to be overfed in the comparison area). At 9 months the infants in the deprived area were found to eat much more chocolate than the others, and less fruit and vegetables (Donnet & Stanfield, 1977).

So, in answer to the question posed earlier, it is perhaps *not* simply a problem of special groups or unusual social circumstances. The general health deficit of children in lower social classes remains clear from the evidence of morbidity and mortality, and it seems unlikely that nutrition plays no part. At this level of general health, however, the clearest evidence can be provided only by children's growth — since it is generally agreed that height is a sensitive measure of nutrition — or by the child-bearing efficiency of women. General social class gradients in the height of children, or in birthweights, are clear and well-known: Tables 13 and 14 return to Scottish figures (Brotherston, 1979).

Table 13. *Height of children by social class, cm, at 14 years, Scotland. From Brotherston (1979)*

Social class	M	F
I	158	156
II	156	156
III	155	155
IV	154	154
V	152	153

Table 14. *Mean birth weight by social class, Scotland, 1971–73. From Brotherston (1979)*

Social class	Birthweight (g)
I	3360
II	3340
III	3270
IV	3240
V	3170

Of course, these measures are strongly influenced by heredity. Many analyses have been made of the relative contributions of biological and social factors in the growth of children — for example that reported by Rona, Swan & Altman (1978) which surveyed the height of children in 22 areas in England and six in Scotland. Differences in height were found to be most closely associated with mother's and father's height (8.4 per cent and 7 per cent of variance respectively) and with birthweight and mother's age. Social class and sibship size accounted for less of the variance, but as Fig. 1 shows, these inter-related variables produced a clear trend by social class. Size of family — in England but not in Scotland — affected height *only* in the manual social classes, except for very large families. This could mean, the authors suggested, that sibship size is associated with height through economic factors, and if there is no hardship the differences apparently attributable to sibship size are partially eliminated.

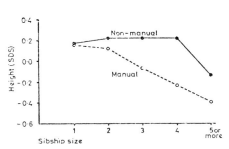

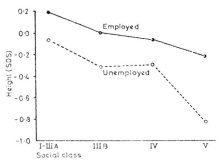

Fig. 1. *Height of children in England expressed in standard deviation score (SDS) according to the occupational status of their fathers and sibship size. (From Rona, Swan & Altman, 1978).*

Fig. 2. *Height of children in England expressed in standard deviation score (SDS) according to social class and employment (or unemployment) of their fathers. (From Rona, Swan & Altman, 1978).*

In this study an interesting relationship was also shown between the father's unemployment and the height of the children. In Scotland, this was stronger than the association with social class.

Obviously, what emerges is a complex of social and biological variables, all associated. Very young mothers of short stature, themselves poorly nourished, are more likely to be in lower social classes (they are also more likely to smoke). They are more likely to have children of low birthweight who are not breast-fed and who are brought up in less than optimum circumstances. Cumulatively, the effects upon development can be large: in the National Child Development Survey, the average difference between those children in the most adverse groups, and those in the most advantageous, was 13.8 cm at seven years (Davie *et al.*, 1972).

D. The meaning of social class

To summarise the argument so far: it has been suggested that there *are* a large number of people in poverty in Britain today, however it is measured, and many of them are mothers and children. Evidence of frank nutritional deficiency is lacking, except in special groups. But the relevance of social class is not simply a likelihood of being at subsistence level in income, because the true meaning of social class is not simply occupational status and its associated income, but an amalgam of life-styles, behaviours and circumstances. When asked

'What decides what class you're in?' nearly half of Townsend's respondents replied, not occupation or income, but 'way of life' or 'family' (Townsend, 1979).

It may be that relatively few, at least among families with children, are actually without the resources nowadays to purchase adequate food. But poverty may be defined in other terms. The consumer goods included in Table 15 are all relevant to the ease and efficiency with which food can be purchased or a household managed. It is well known that poorer families spend a higher proportion of their income upon food, but less often realised that the proportion of income spent on necessities may be rising, rather than falling. It is usually thought that

Table 15. *Ownership of goods. (General Household Survey, 1979)*

	% Not owning:		
	Refrigerator	Telephone	Car
Head of household			
Professional	2	6	10
Employers and managerial	3	9	15
Intermediate non-manual	4	17	32
Junior non-manual	4	20	47
Skilled manual	5	30	38
Semi-skilled manual, service	7	43	65
Unskilled manual	9	56	80

the *greater* amount than the median on fuel, light and heat represents inefficient and expensive heating systems. Certainly there is little indication here of what Rowntree called 'secondary poverty', or the situation where an income would provide for adequate subsistence, if it were not spent on non-essentials.

As Donnison (1981) has noted, many of those living near subsistence level

'. . . dull their appetites with cigarettes, cups of tea, biscuits and sticky buns. Some — poorly fed and ill-clad — burn far too much electricity keeping themselves warm. But their problems are unlikely to be solved by lectures on domestic science.'

In making this final point, some evidence is offered from a study of the health of children in a sample of 58 families in social classes IV and V in Aberdeen (Blaxter & Paterson, 1982). This was not a nutritional

Table 16. *Comparative expenditure 1953-73 of families in 5th percentile of incomes. From Fiegelen et al. (1977)*

	Expenditure as % of median	
	1953	1973
Housing	63	70
Fuel light power	100	114
Food	72	72
Alcoholic drink	53	33
Durables	43	52
Transport, vehicles	33	23

survey, and there is no detailed information on the children's diets. Observation and discussion during a close association with the families over six months suggested, however, that diets in the poorest families were certainly not optimal. In part, this was due to poor nutritional knowledge. A quotation from the transcripts of tape-recorded interviews may demonstrate this:

'I took rickets as a child — nobody else in the family took rickets, I don't know why I took it, I could have been playing with someone who had it and passed it on.'

This also gives some indication of the typically poor health history of the young mothers themselves, which was, of course, associated with a poorer perinatal record in the children.

As babies, the children were rarely breast-fed: only nine of the mothers had even attempted breast-feeding, for only 14 of the 139 children. The reasons which they offered were frequently to do with convenience — they were intending to go back to work, the demands of other small children made it too difficult — but many also spoke of it as a 'strange' or repugnant idea:

'You didn't associate your breasts with feeding. They were sort of part of your figure'

or expressed acute embarrassment about it:

'I wouldn't like to do it in front of my own husband, never mind anyone else. I wouldn't do it in front of my sister-in-law, and she comes in every

day. And if a crowd of people came in, you couldn't just sit and breast-
feed, so you'd have to go into another room and everyone would know
why.'

Despite the fact that the promotion of breast-feeding is the formal
policy of maternity hospitals and health visitors, the young mothers did
not describe a great deal of pressure or education about it. On the later
feeding of infants, however, there was continual conflict with health
professionals. The mothers believed firmly in very early weaning or
supplementation; they felt that they 'knew' what their baby wanted,
and if early solids 'cured' a baby of crying all night, this was clear proof
that they were right. Typical accounts were:

'I just put what we're having in the liquidiser. She has all sorts of things
— I like to let her taste lots of different things' (baby of six weeks).

'When I came home from the hospital I put him on full cream and half
a rusk. The health visitor didn't like that! So I stopped telling her. She'd
say, "now, you're only giving him his bottle, aren't you?" And I'd say,
yes, yes!'.

This conflict was obviously harmful to the relationship between the
young mothers and health visitors, and might turn the women against
attending clinics altogether. These findings about breast-feeding and
early weaning, where young mothers in difficult circumstances feel
that the practices recommended to them are simply not appropriate to
their style of living, are of course common ones.

As the children became older, most of the families were observed to
eat, and agreed that they ate, large quantities of tinned food, pies,
icecream, soft drinks, cakes and baker's products generally, with little
fresh meat or vegetables. Some made a point of saying that they gave
fruit to their children, though others claimed that it was too expensive.
These diets were not defended, but they were seen as inevitable, in
their particular circumstances. To these families, the idea of a 'proper'
or family meal was not necessarily appropriate. Single-handed mothers
got into a habit of continual snacks, or the husband's tastes were said to
prevail:

'It's difficult, when it's just you and the kids. You haven't got to make
meat and that, so you don't — you get like them, eating rubbish all the
time'
'Their father eats no vegetables at all, so neither do they'

'I used to make a meal with potatoes at lunch-time, but I stopped because they wouldn't take it'.

Many mothers were working, in some cases in the evenings, so that fathers had to feed and look after the children. Many children had meals at school or day nurseries. If the father was unemployed, it might be he who prepared meals. Different members of the family might be having their main meal at different times, so there were few occasions for a formal family meal.

The idea of a store cupboard or vegetable garden, from which meals might be prepared, was not always appropriate for a young urban generation. Working mothers, or those tied to the house by small children, or those living in housing estates where only 'corner shops' or visiting vans were easily accessible, naturally tended towards a pattern of piecemeal shopping, buying food to eat immediately. Only a few of these families did weekly shopping at supermarkets, for this would imply the use of a car, and would certainly involve the laying-out of larger sums of money at one time. Small local shops tended largely to stock packeted and tinned goods, in small sizes, and a vicious circle was set up: this was what was easily available, so the families bought it; this was what they bought, so it was stocked in the shops. The resultant diet may have been nutritionally adequate, but it certainly represented inefficient spending.

With the exception of milk, which the mothers did emphasise as important for their children, the cheapest and most basic foods — bread, porridge, the home-made soup that had been the pride of a thrifty older generation — seemed to have about them an association with poverty and the 'bad old days'. One mother, for instance, said that she was ashamed because her child liked to eat bread

'. . . with nothing on it. I'm affronted in case anyone sees her. She doesn't even fold it over'.

Such things as cake, icecream, tinned fruit, on the other hand, represented the ability to buy things which had been rare luxuries in their own childhood. To find it difficult to restrict children's sweet-eating is a common enough experience in all families, but for these there were special pressures towards indulgence: as one mother explained, very simply, her husband

'. . . gives them sweets because he never got, and he doesn't want them to do without'.

The families also had to deal with a special hazard — the travelling vans which toured the estates, offering continual temptation:

'One icecream van comes round three times of an evening — she wants something from every van that comes'.

Thus cultural, commercial, and practical pressures dictated dietary habits. Regional patterns of eating will always be a complicating factor in the consideration of diets, and one cannot necessarily generalise from one small and local study. It is only at this intensive level, however, that the real consequences of poverty in behavioural terms can be demonstrated. This study suggested that poverty can be defined in terms of constraints upon choice, and powerlessness over the environment. In the circumstances of deprived lives, certain behaviours — from early childbearing to patterns of eating — are inevitable. The 'culture of poverty' is a concept now largely discredited, if it implies simply persisting subcultural beliefs and behaviours. However, the very practical constraints of poverty remain.

References

Benson, P. F., Stroud, C. E., Mitchell, N. J. & Nicolaides, A. (1963): Rickets in immigrant children in Glasgow. *British Medical Journal* 1, 1054.

Berthoud, R., Brown, J. C. & Cooper, S. (1981): *Poverty and the Development of Anti-poverty in the UK*. London: Heinemann.

Beveridge, W. (1942): *Social Insurance and Allied Services*. London: HMSO.

Blaxter, M. & Paterson, E. (1982): *Mothers and Daughters*. London: Heinemann Educational Books.

Brotherston, Sir J. (1979): Inequality, is it inevitable? In *Equalities and Inequalities in Health*, ed C. O. Carter & J. Peel. London: Academic Press.

Community Relations Commission (1977): Evidence to the Royal Commission on the National Health Service.

Davie, R., Butler, N. & Goldstein, H. (1972): *From Birth to Seven*. London: Longman.

Donnet, M. L. & Stanfield, J. P. (1977): A survey of infant nutrition, growth and development in Glasgow. *Nutrition and Metabolism* 21, Suppl. 1.

Donnison, D. (1981): *The Politics of Poverty*. London: Martin Robertson.

Exton-Smith, A. N. (1979): Eating habits of the elderly. In *Nutrition and Lifestyles*, ed M. R. Turner. London: Applied Science.

Fiegehen, G. C., Lansley, P. S. & Smith, A. D. (1977): *Poverty and Progress in Britain 1953–73*. Cambridge: Cambridge University Press.

General Household Survey (1979): London: HMSO.

Goel, K. M. (1979): Nutrition Survey of Immigrant Children in Glasgow. *Scottish Health Service Studies* No. 40. Edinburgh: Scottish Home and Health Department.

Goel, K. M., Campbell, S., Logan, R. W., Sweet, E. M., Attenburrow, A. & Arneil, G. C. (1981): Reduced prevalence of rickets in Asian children in Glasgow. *Lancet* 1, 405.

Kincaid, J. C. (1975): *Poverty and Equality in Britain*. Harmondsworth: Penguin.

Lawson, D. E. M., Paul, A. A. & Black, A. E. (1979): Relative contributions of diet and sunlight to vitamin D status in the elderly. *British Medical Journal* 2, 303.

Layard, R., Piachaud, D. & Stewart, M. (1978): The Causes of Poverty. Background Paper No. 5, Royal Commission on the Distribution of Income and Wealth. London: HMSO.

Manchester Community Health Group for Ethnic Minorities (1980): Rickets in Britain.

Pearson, D., Burns, S. & Cunningham, K. (1977): Dietary surveys of immigrant schoolgirls in Leicester. *Journal of Human Nutrition* 31, 362.

Richards, I. D. G., Sweet, E. M. & Arneil, G. C. (1968): Infantile rickets persists in Glasgow. *Lancet* 1, 803.

Rona, R. J., Swan, A. V. & Altman, D. G. (1978): Social factors and height of primary school children in England and Scotland. *Journal of Epidemiology and Community Health* 32, 147.

Rowntree, Seerbohm (1901): *Poverty: A Study of Town Life*. London: Macmillan.

Rowntree, Seerbohm (1937): *The Human Needs of Labour*. London: Longman.

Ruck, N. (1979): Social influences on the diets of immigrant families. In *Nutrition and Lifestyles*, ed M. R. Turner. London: Applied Science.

Townsend, P. (1979): *Poverty in the United Kingdom*. Harmondsworth: Penguin.

Walker, C. L. & Church, M. (1978): Poverty by administration: a review of Supplementary Benefits, nutrition, and scale rates. *Journal of Human Nutrition* 32, 5.

3

Trends in meal planning and eating habits

STEPHEN KING

A. Introduction

William Harrison's 'A Description of England', published in 1577, gives us a fair idea of what townspeople ate in Tudor times. They had three meals a day — breakfast, a midday meal and supper. At the midday meal, for instance, they might have soup, then stew or pie or roast meat with onions, then bread and cheese, all washed down with ale. The meal was often eaten at a tavern or bought at a cookshop and taken home. There was a good deal less variety in vegetables than we have today and fruit and sweet pastries were rather occasional treats. But, otherwise, William Harrison might have been writing about the 1980s. There have been massive changes in the way that food has been preserved and packed, but it is easy to get the impression that nothing very much has changed over 400 years in meal planning and eating habits. In this chapter I want to examine the published evidence for the stability of food choice over the past 20 years and for more recent changes, then to speculate about what lies behind those changes.

B. Stability in choice of food

The broadest way in which we can look at people's choice in the home is to see how the weekly budget is spent on the main categories of food. Fortunately we have the long series of the National Food Survey to allow us to do this with reasonable accuracy. Table 1 shows the changes between the first five years of the 1960s and the last five years of the 1970s. Share of the weekly food budget spent on meat has increased quite markedly, by 3 percentage points, and on vegetables has grown by 1 percentage point. Eggs have declined quite sharply in share, cereal products (mainly bread) and sugar a little. But the overwhelming impression is one of stability. After fifteen years of what often seems to be marked social and economic turbulence there is

Table 1. *Share of domestic food expenditure. (MAFF: National Food Survey)*

	All households		
	Average 1960-64 (%)	Average 1975-79 (%)	Difference
Dairy products	16.6	16.3	*
Margarine & other fats	2.1	2.1	*
Meat	28.5	31.5	+3.0
Cereals	15.3	14.8	−0.5
Vegetables	11.2	12.2	+1.0
Fruit	6.3	5.9	*
Fish	4.4	4.2	*
Eggs	4.7	3.0	−1.7
Sugar & preserves	3.6	2.7	−0.9
Beverages & misc	7.4	7.3	*
	100	100	

* = less than 0.5 percentage points

nothing *fundamentally* different about the way in which the household food budget is spent. Roughly two-and-a-half times as much is still spent on meat as on vegetables, and about one-sixth of weekly spending still goes on dairy products.

This apparent conservatism goes further than stability over time. We can get an idea of how pervasive the pattern is by looking at the same breakdown for different groups of the population. For instance, Table 2 compares with the all-household average the spending of households containing two adults only and those containing two adults and two children. Not surprisingly, the differences in the sheer amount spent on food are quite considerable — the adult households spending about 40 per cent more per head than the adults-plus-children households. But within the totals the differences in the way that the money is spent are really quite small. The biggest divergence is for meat, which takes up a larger than average share of budget for the adult families and a smaller than average share for the adults-plus-children. But in each case the difference is under 2 percentage points.

I have looked in exactly the same way at divergences from the norm by head of household's gross earnings, by housing tenure, by household income and by region, and the picture is always much the same (BNF, 1981). In none of the cases examined was the difference greater than 2 percentage points for any of the ten main food categories. Regional

Table 2. *Share of domestic food expenditure. (MAFF: National Food Survey)*

Difference in percentage points from all households, 1979

	2-adult households	2-adult + 2-children households
Dairy products	− 0.8	+ 0.8
Margarine & other fats	*	*
Meat	+ 1.9	− 1.6
Cereals	− 1.5	+ 1.1
Vegetables	− 0.6	*
Fruit	*	*
Fish	+ 0.5	*
Eggs	*	*
Sugar & preserves	*	*
Beverages & misc	*	*

* = less than 0.5 percentage points

differences were as large as any, and were very persistent over time. This is not to suggest that there have been no changes in the food that people eat. There are very marked differences between consumption today and consumption pre-war, and even within the post-rationing period the decline of bread and potatoes and the growth of meat have been considerable. At the same time there can be big individual variations within broad groups of people.

Nevertheless, compared to other areas of spending, the food market appears to have been unusually stable and slow-moving. The way in which people choose to spend their weekly budget has been remarkably consistent over time and within group. It suggests that the prime determinant of meal planning and eating habits has been the culture in which we live, the ideas about the proper way to behave that are handed down from generation to generation and are reflected in the popular media.

But so far I have been looking at how the money is spent, rather than what is got for it, and I have taken five-year averages to measure change in the last two decades. Lurking under these averages are some sharp recent changes in consumption, with very important implications.

C. The new discontinuities

1. Eating in

Even taking share of domestic food expenditure, it is clear that there was something of a watershed in 1970. Between 1960 and 1970 the

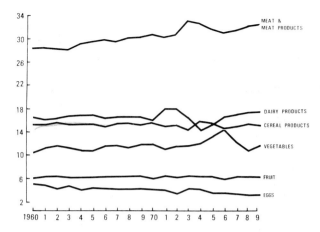

Fig. 1. *Share of domestic food expenditure according to main food
categories, 1960–69. (MAFF: National Food Survey)*

Table 3. *Range of annual consumptions (oz per head/week). (MAFF:
National Food Survey)*

	Index: 100 = 1970 household consumption					
	1960–1970 (Indices of consumption)		*1970–1980 (Indices of consumption)*		*Range of consumption (index points)*	
	Lowest	*Highest*	*Lowest*	*Highest*	*1960s*	*1970s*
Dairy products						
Liquid milk	100	106	94	106	6	12
Cheese	85	100	99	108	15	9
Butter	95	104	68	100	9	32
Margarine & other fats	93	106	91	120	13	29
Meat						
Carcase meat & chicken	92	102	95	112	10	17
Cereal products						
Bread	99	119	81	100	20	19
All other cereals	97	101	88	100	4	12
Vegetables	94	101	79	100	7	21
Potatoes	95	107	66	100	12	34
Fruit	94	103	94	110	9	16
Fish	100	111	77	100	11	23
Eggs	95	102	81	100	7	19
Sugar & preserves	97	111	68	100	14	32
Beverages						
Tea	97	110	77	100	13	23
Coffee	68	102	84	119	34	35

shares for each of the main categories were very stable from year to year; the patterns of change were very smooth. After 1970 there started to be quite marked fluctuations, as Fig. 1 shows.

These discontinuities were very much greater in terms of absolute amounts consumed. Table 3 demonstrates this by indexing the consumption of 15 commodities, noting the high and low points, and hence the range of consumption in each decade. Of the 15 categories listed, 12 show markedly greater variations in the 1970s than in the 1960s: roughly double the range. Of the exceptions, bread shows a steady decline in consumption in both decades; cheese a steady growth, but rather slower in the 1970s; coffee a slower growth in the 1970s, but with much more violent fluctuations.

Figure 2 shows the typical pattern. For each year between 1960 and 1970 consumption per head of carcase meat, fish, eggs and potatoes lay within ±10 per cent of the 1970 figure, but thereafter the range was far wider. On the whole, the more these broad categories are broken down into component parts, the more violent the fluctuations. To take two quite extreme (but in my view significant) cases, consumption of cakes and pastries went down 9 per cent in the 1960s and 38 per cent in the 1970s; while consumption of ice cream mousse and soufflé went up 39 per cent in the 1960s and 184 per cent in the 1970s. There is every indication that the former solidity of the food culture started to break down after 1970.

But the National Food Survey covers domestic consumption only. Though published data on eating out are, by comparison, very sketchy, it seems that recent change there has been even greater.

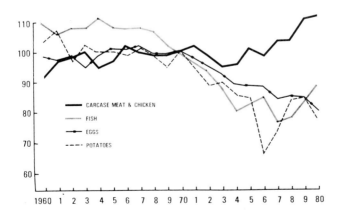

Fig. 2. *Domestic food consumption in ounces per head per week (Index: 100 = 1970) of some principal food categories. (MAFF: National Food Survey)*

2. Eating out

There has been a fairly steady increase in the sheer amount of eating out over the last 20 years. In 1960, according to the Family Expenditure Survey, meals taken out of the home accounted for 9.7 per cent of total expenditure on food; by 1970 it was 13.5 per cent, and in 1979 16.4 per cent. The National Food Survey gives much less data, but in recent years has noted the number of meals taken out per person per week. Between 1973 and 1979 midday meals out rose from 1.66 per person per week to 1.81 (that is, + 9 per cent) and other meals out — surely evening meals for the most part — rose from 1.03 to 1.39 (+ 35 per cent).

There are far greater differences between households in eating out than in eating in, particularly in terms of household income. To illustrate this, Table 4 compares three groups of households. The first had low incomes (£40–50 per week in 1979), the second medium incomes (£120–140 per week) and the third high incomes (over £250 per week). There is relatively little difference between the three groups in terms of expenditure per head on food eaten in, and a good deal of that difference can be explained by household composition. The low earners tend to be older and without children; the medium earners have a high ratio of children to adults; the high earners have a high proportion of wage-earners. Despite these marked differences in type of household, the breakdown of the domestic food budget is strikingly similar. (The percentages in the Family Expenditure Survey are different from those in the National Food Survey, since its miscellaneous category also covers sweets, chocolates and soft drinks). But there are massive differences in money spent on eating out. As a result, the high-earning households spent only 11 per cent more per head than the low-earning on food in the home, but 38 per cent more on food in total.

There are also quite marked regional variations in eating out, which seem related to urban/rural differences. In East Anglia and the South West, for instance, meals out accounted for 13.6 per cent of food expenditure in 1978–9; in the West Midlands it was 15.3 per cent; and in Greater London 19.8 per cent. Once again, these relationships between regions seem very stable over time.

Two fairly clear conclusions emerge. First, as the tendency to eat out is so firmly correlated with household income, we can expect the trend to continue as real household income rises. Secondly, the apparent stability of breakdown of the domestic food budget by category may be giving us a misleading impression. If, as seems likely, what people eat

Table 4. *Household food expenditure, 1979. (DOE: Family Expenditure Survey)*

	Households with gross normal weekly income of:		
	£40–50 (%)	£120–140 (%)	Over £250 (%)
Expenditure on food eaten in:			
Dairy products	15.9	15.6	15.1
Margarine & other fats	2.2	1.8	1.5
Meat	28.8	27.4	30.4
Cereals	14.2	14.1	12.2
Vegetables	9.3	10.2	9.7
Fruit	5.1	5.2	6.3
Fish	4.7	4.4	4.4
Eggs	2.9	2.3	2.2
Sugar & preserves	3.1	1.9	1.7
Beverages & misc.	13.6	17.0	16.5
	100	100	100
Indices of expenditure per head on:			
(100 = expenditure of £40–50 group per head)			
Food eaten in	94	91	105
Food eaten out	6	18	33
Total	100	109	138
Household composition			
Adults under retirement age	0.8	1.9	2.8
Adults over retirement age	0.9	0.1	0.1
Children	0.3	1.1	1.0
	1.95	3.13	3.87

out is different from what they eat in, eating habits are changing somewhat faster than the National Food Survey suggests.

Unfortunately, neither of the basic continuous sources gives us any data about what it is that people eat out. The main published survey has been carried out by Gallup, first for the Hotels and Catering Economic Development Council (1974–77) and more recently under the title of 'The British survey of eating out' (Social Surveys [Gallup Poll] Ltd, 1978–). While this is valuable information, the survey has been running only seven years and, for various reasons, cannot give

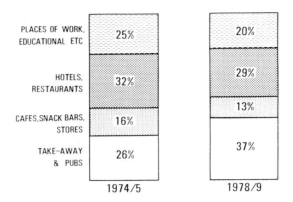

PLACES OF WORK,
EDUCATIONAL ETC   25%   20%

HOTELS,
RESTAURANTS   32%   29%

                                      13%
CAFES, SNACK BARS,
STORES   16%

TAKE-AWAY   37%
& PUBS   26%

          1974/5   1978/9

Fig. 3. *Share of expenditure on meals out according to where meal was eaten.*
(Social Surveys [Gallup Poll] Ltd)

a great deal of detail. However, even within these limitations, it shows
a very dramatic change in the catering outlets in which people spend
their money (see Fig. 3). Share of expenditure accounted for by pubs
and take-away restaurants is shown as rising from 26 per cent to 37 per
cent between 1974/5 and 1978/9, and it seems highly likely that this
trend has continued. Over half the meals eaten out were defined by the
eaters as 'snacks' rather than 'main meals'. This is confirmed by the
Target Group Index, a very large-scale continuous consumer survey,
which shows that the proportion of adults who buy take-away food rose
from 33 per cent in 1974 to 57 per cent in 1981. The figures for the
under-35s are even more striking — from 52 per cent to 80 per cent in
the same seven years. The implication is very strong that not only is
food eaten out different from food eaten in, but it is changing more
rapidly.

D. What lies behind the changes?

We are left therefore with very strong evidence that the old stabilities
of British eating habits have been, and are increasingly, breaking
down. We have a fair amount of information about *the ways* in which
they are breaking down, although the information is decidedly patchy
when we try to relate the food eaten out to the food eaten in. But we
are desperately short of data to explain *why* it is all happening or what
lies behind these changes and discontinuities. This means that, at the
moment, we have to use a great deal of judgement and speculation in

order to pick out likely trends in the future. Simply projecting past consumption trends will hardly be very successful, if the figures are fluctuating violently from year to year. At the same time, we face a situation in which there is likely to be increasing concern from official bodies and pressure groups about 'healthy eating', with attempts to influence public opinion. These attempts are likely to be either ineffective or counter-productive if the would-be influencers do not understand why eating patterns are changing.

Happily, the British Nutrition Foundation and some of its members are now undertaking a programme of consumer research to make a start on bridging the information gaps. Meanwhile, we can raise hypotheses about what lies behind the new discontinuities and test them against what is known now. Quite clearly, the answers are going to be complex; there will be no simple solution. But I would like here to examine three of the main ideas about what is causing eating habits to change.

1. The price hypothesis

The most obvious potential cause is inflation. Not only was the rate of inflation much higher in the 1970s than in the 1960s, but so also were the variations from year to year in *real prices* — that is, in prices relative to those of the Retail Price Index for food. Table 5 shows the range of real prices for 16 food categories in the 1960s and 1970s, calculated in the same way as in Table 3. In only two cases — poultry and bread — were the variations in real price less in the 1970s than in the 1960s. In most of the rest, the differences were substantial.

There is undoubtedly evidence to support the hypothesis that fluctuations in prices have been responsible for some of the new discontinuities in consumption. This is of course particularly so when price increases have been unusually great: for instance, with coffee in 1977, sugar in 1975 and 1976 or potatoes in 1976. There are whole categories of food for which, it seems, the 'economist's rules' apply: that is, consumption goes up when real prices go down, and vice versa. For instance, when annual fish consumption is indexed and plotted against the inverse of the index of real price for fish, the two lines are very nearly coincident for 20 years (Fig. 4). The same is true for carcase meat in the 1960s; it is broadly true for the 1970s, though the fit is less good. Beyond these instances, the price hypothesis looks fairly vulnerable. The price and consumption lines for poultry are quite close in the 1960s, but the fit is poor in the 1970s: consumption carried on growing, while real price stabilised. In the same way, bread continued

Table 5. *Range of annual real prices. (MAFF: National Food Survey)*

	1960s (index points)	1970s (index points)
Dairy products		
Liquid milk	7	33
Cheese	9	30
Butter	31	44
Margarine	15	20
Meat		
Carcase meat	15	21
Poultry	51	9
Cereal products		
Bread	27	12
All other cereals	4	15
Vegetables	16	40
Potatoes	38	138
Fruit	9	12
Fish	8	22
Eggs	29	30
Sugar	30	90
Preserves	10	23
Beverages	27	54

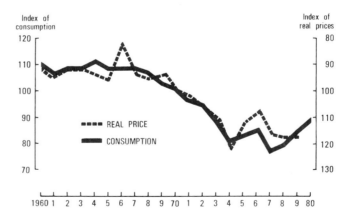

Fig. 4. *Consumption of fish compared with real price: ounces per head per week vs prices deflated by Retail Price Index for food: Index: 100 = 1970. (MAFF: National Food Survey)*

to decline, while real price stabilised. And for eggs and cheese, after a reasonably close fit in the 1960s, the lines are actually going in the 'wrong' direction in the 1970s. Consumption of eggs declined by 20 per cent, while their real price also declined by 20 per cent (Fig. 5). Cheese consumption steadily increased, despite real price increases of up to 30 per cent and very sharp fluctuations (Fig. 6). It seems fairly clear that poultry and cheese have some sort of 'added values' that are the main causes of changes in their consumption, and bread and eggs have

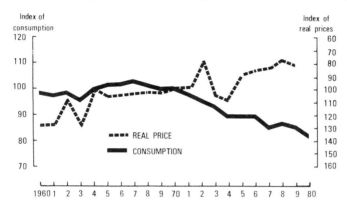

Fig. 5. *Consumption of eggs compared with real price: number per head per week vs prices deflated by Retail Price Index for food: Index: 100 = 1970. (MAFF: National Food Survey)*

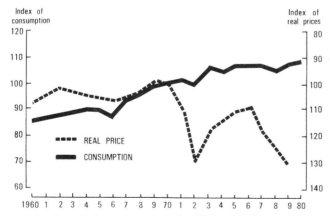

Fig. 6. *Consumption of cheese compared with real price: ounces per head per week vs prices deflated by Retail Price Index for food: Index: 100 = 1970. (MAFF: National Food Survey)*

some sort of 'diminished values'. In fact, a good deal of analysis and market modelling has been done on bread, and the trends which emerge as having the closest correlation are bread consumption and the inverse of real personal disposable income. That is, as people become better off, they eat less bread. The implications of this finding are supported by consumer attitude research, which shows that while brown bread is very highly respected, bread generally, and white bread in particular, has been looked on as a cheap filler. It seems likely that bread has suffered through being seen as too cheap or as 'cheap and nasty'. By contrast, frozen peas have steadily gained share of market at the expense of canned peas, despite a price premium of anything from 50 per cent to 200 per cent.

This is, of course, to look at food in the home only. The price hypothesis seems to explain even less outside the home. It is hard to believe that people are increasingly eating out in order to save money, particularly as the cost of meals out has risen faster than that of food in general over the last five years. Relative price is likely to have been involved in the move from traditional cafes to take-away, fast food and pub meals, but it seems doubtful whether it has been the major factor.

In general, therefore, we can conclude that fluctuations in price have had some effect in changing eating habits. But they do not seem to explain very much; there are several instances where the price hypothesis would be actively misleading; on the whole, relative price seems less important than it used to be.

2. The healthy eating hypothesis

Another hypothesis put forward is that there has been a marked increase in the desire for 'healthy eating' and that this is beginning to affect people's habits. There is indeed a fair amount of incidental evidence for this from consumer research in certain markets. For instance, there is a belief among some people, in a rather vague way, that there is some sort of relationship between polyunsaturated fats, cholesterol, blood pressure, heart attacks and low-fat spreads. The ideas that lie behind the beliefs may be somewhat unformed or confused, but they are certainly having some effect on the choice of brands and types of spread. Equally, many people interested in nutrition have been encouraged by, say, the growth in margarine consumption at the expense of butter, or in the rapid gains for wholemeal bread, or in the decline in cake consumption. They feel this to be a sign that the public is putting its ideas on nutrition into practice. However, the healthy eating hypothesis does not stand up to much examination. There is depressingly little information on what the public believes, but there is a fair amount on what people do. Over the years the National Food Survey has been calculating the proportions of total energy derived from protein, fat and carbohydrate in food eaten at home. Although there is room for doubts about the absolute figures and means of measurement, the trends have been consistent and unequivocal. Fig. 7 shows the 1960 and 1979 figures.

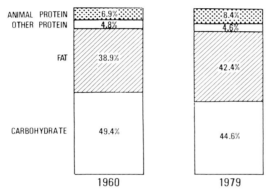

Fig. 7. *The nutritional value of household food: a comparison of the proportions of total energy derived from protein, fat and carbohydrate of food eaten at home between 1960 and 1979. (MAFF: National Food Survey)*

A steadily higher proportion of energy has come from fat and animal protein, at the expense of carbohydrate. In that the process has gone further with the better-off, there is every reason to believe that the trend will continue. Yet there is an almost universal consensus that this is an undesirable direction. Dietary guidelines that have been proposed (DHSS, 1979; Turner & Gray, 1982) clearly advocate a reduction in consumption of fat and alcohol (which has also been increasing) and an increase in carbohydrates. We can say that, if it is in fact a desire for healthy eating that is affecting eating habits, something is going rather badly wrong.

The information currently available does not allow us to be certain whether people genuinely do want to eat in a more healthy way, but have misunderstood how to do so; whether they are merely paying lip-service to the idea; or whether it is an issue that rarely crosses their minds. We badly need consumer research data of the sort that the BNF is now collecting.

Meanwhile it is possible, by putting together pieces of information from various sources (BNF, 1981), to get a reasonably consistent, if tentative, picture of public attitudes to eating and health. The evidence is that people have become increasingly familiar with nutritional terms, and are reasonably able to associate them with specific foods. Meat, eggs, cheese and fish are associated with protein; butter, milk, cheese and meat with fats; bread and potatoes with both carbohydrates and calories. Butter and eggs are for some people associated wtih cholesterol; breakfast cereals (especially bran cereals) — and occasionally vegetables — with dietary fibre. But, however sensible people's views are, the research tends to suggest that the level of knowledge is fairly superficial.

Various surveys have shown that there is a broad but partial awareness of the roles of nutrients, with certain gaps — for instance, little mention of fruit and vegetables for roughage — and certain misconceptions — for instance, the association of calories and 'fattening'. People's knowledge is rather firmer when they are questioned on the roles of foods rather than of nutrients. For instance, when asked to name foods for 'body-building in growing children' they tend to pick out foods which are in fact high in protein. Fruit and vegetables are rated consistently well, even though few people are clear of how they fit into the process of nutrition. Bread and potatoes tend to be rated lower than they deserve, at least partly because of their associations with 'fattening'; but otherwise general knowledge on the role of foods seems quite reasonable. However, there is a good deal of circumstantial evidence that a lot of this knowledge is not being used. This is partly because it has not been received in a usable form and partly because it has not been properly linked with the emotional and sensual pleasures people get from food.

First and perhaps most important, knowledge of nutrients is of little values to people if they do not know how to relate it to the choices that they have to make in their daily lives — which are about successions of meals, amounts and choice within categories. There appears to be a strong emotional involvement in the idea of a balanced diet, but very few people are able to define what is meant by a balanced diet. On the whole, it is seen as meaning a varied diet, concentrating on the foods that are 'good for you' and trying not to have too much of foods that are 'bad for you'. Secondly, there is a great deal of irritated scepticism about the specific nutritional ideas that people come across. This is because 'the experts' seem either to express their views forcibly, but contradict each other, or they hedge their bets by making the whole topic very complicated. Two people who expressed this irritation in recent group discussions were summing up a very prevalent view. One said 'On the one hand, you're told it's good for you and on the other hand you read it isn't good for you. One minute it's giving you protein; the next it's making you fat.' The other said: 'You don't know what to believe these days. They're always getting at you.' Thirdly, because so often awareness of the importance of nutrition has been linked with self-denial and has been presented as an intellectual exercise, it is not a very attractive idea to many people. It has become divorced from the pleasures of eating, and people are made to feel guilty when the subject arises. As the researcher in one survey (Kraft, 1978) put it: 'The trouble with the word "nutrition" is that it is too often directly associated with unpleasant activities such as slimming or illness, rather than pleasurable ones. Also, it has a rather "medical" or "chemical" ring to it'.

Table 6. *How people normally find out 'what's good for you'. (Kraft survey, 1978)*

Percent saying:	Women (%)	Men (%)
Common sense	64	53
Magazines, newspapers	37	27
Books	29	32
Family	24	34
Doctor	18	11
TV	16	21
Friends	13	10
School	9	4

As a result, people seem to turn away from what knowledge they have and look for simple rules — such as that fresh or natural foods (including frozen foods) are better for you than processed, or that carbohydrates are fattening (so cut down on them when you're overweight, and everything will be all right). This approach was illustrated well (Kraft, 1978) when people were asked how they normally find out what's good for you. Table 6 shows the answers. Common sense emerged as overwhelmingly the most important source; then informal learning from the entertainment media; with books, probably specifically on diets, next; and doctors and teachers (the 'experts') a rather bad fourth. This sort of attitude makes it hard to give much weight to the healthy eating hypothesis. There may well be some increasing interest in healthy eating, but with so much muddle, scepticism and desire for commonsense solutions, it is difficult to see how it could be responsible for much of the new discontinuities in eating habits.

3. The social change hypothesis

The third hypothesis is that finally the social change which has affected so many other aspects of life — work, leisure, the home, attitudes to authority, dress and so on — is beginning to change that most conservative of habits, eating. One of the main changes in people's attitudes over the last twenty years or so can be summed up as the *new individualism*. There has been something of a revolution in responses to authorities, institutions and organisations, based on a desire for personal freedom and a realisation that it is attainable. People have been moving from fixed and inherited values to individual and discovered values. There has been a strong feeling that 'everything's getting too big', an antagonism to the producer bureaucracy and an unwillingness to accept the ideas of authorities without question. People's horizons have broadened in many ways, but particularly in a desire for self-expression and self-determination.

There are indications of this new individualism throughout British society. The 'women's movement' is one of the more obvious manifestations; for instance, the proportion of married women who have jobs has risen considerably and is the highest in Europe. Perhaps more important, there is direct research evidence that this has widened their perceptions of their roles: more today see themselves as working people who also run a house rather than housewives who also have a job. Ownership of homes has doubled in the last 30 years, of cars in the last 20 years — both aspects of individualism, having one's own private space. Education — developing the ability to work out one's own views (in theory, anyhow) — has boomed: twice as many of the under-thirties get O-Levels as did their parents' generation. Just as significant, there has also been a boom in informal education — watching television, reading specialist magazines, visiting museums and art galleries, attending evening classes and travelling abroad.

The new individualism has been fuelled by the growth in real disposable income: consumer expenditure has gone up by about 25 per cent in real terms in each of the last two decades. We often seem to ignore this increase in affluence, for two reasons. First, because the media concentrate on the bad economic news, which tends to be dramatic, rather than the good, which tends to be gradual. Secondly, because economic advance is by no means universal, relative deprivation is, if anything, becoming a worse problem. The situation was well described by Richard Bourne (1979), after exposure to the survey work of Dr Halsey and his associates, as 'a growing but increasingly hetero-geneous middle class underpinned by an increasingly tight, self-recruited working class'. Very properly, there is a good deal of concentration on those who are not participating in the new individualism. For those interested in nutrition, the pockets of inadequate eating have been the traditional area for study, but it is clear that if the 'diseases of affluence' are growing in importance, we shall have to pay more attention to the majority. The evidence that the new individualism has been affecting eating habits is inevitably circumstantial, but cumulatively there is quite a lot of it and it all seems to point in the same direction.

Perhaps a starting point is to look at how people have been spending their money on things for the home. Table 7 shows the changes in ownership in the 1970s. It is clear that the pattern is different from the 1960s. The more functional sort of goods — like vacuum cleaners, irons, washing machines and refrigerators — have more or less reached saturation point. Though there will be a certain amount of replace-ment and upgrading, there is no longer the pressure for first acquisition. (Interestingly, this seems to be true also for cars.) The major areas of growth in the 1970s were for durables offering enter-tainment and social life — in particular, colour television and the telephone, and there seems little doubt that in the 1980s the growth will come in videotape recorders and other sorts of electronic entertain-ment. It is one of a number of indications that people are moving from goods to services and that social relationships are proliferating. Two items of kitchen equipment feature in the list — freezers and food mixers. Although there is no direct evidence, it seems likely that both

Table 7. *Changes in ownership in the 1970s. (BMRB: Target Group Index)*

Per cent of households owning:	1971 (%)	1981 (%)	Change
Colour TV	3	69	+ 66
Telephone	37	77	+ 40
Separate deep freeze	3	31	+ 28
Food mixer	30	52	+ 22
Full central heating	12	31	+ 19
Refrigerator or fridge/freezer	70	89	+ 19
Car	55	64	+ 9
Washing machine	68	76	+ 8
Vacuum cleaner	85	83	− 2

will be affecting cooking styles and kitchen traditions, particularly the mixers. This is confirmed by research (BMRB, 1978) which shows that, while the use of recipes for cakes and puddings has grown only a little, the proportion of women using them for main dishes rose from 15 per cent in 1961 to 49 per cent in 1977. Qualitative research suggests that this has been accompanied by a change in the perceived role of different foods. Twenty years ago the aesthetic and sensual aspects of cakes and puddings were seen as particularly important, but for main dishes the more functional aspects of being 'nutritious' and 'filling' predominated. Today there is a much greater inclination to see the role of *all* cooking as to give pleasure, to express creativity and to communicate.

The first (qualitative) stages of the new BNF survey have picked out a fascinating difference in the generations. The researcher commented that among middle-aged respondents in the North it sometimes appeared that the washing-up was the main point of an evening meal. There was a strong desire to eat early, so as to get the washing-up done early. Several of those interviewed expressed some concern about visiting their married offspring who gave them a meal mid-evening, and indeed often lingered over it. One respondent described such behaviour as 'degenerate'. The offspring tended to see the evening meal much more as an aesthetic or expressive activity. In such circumstances, it is hardly surprising that the number of visits by older relatives has not gone up over the years (JWT, 1981). But the proportion of under-35 housewives who had received visits from friends in the last week went up from 52 per cent to 66 per cent between 1965 and 1980. While there are no reliable trend data available, if we rely on people's own ideas of how their habits have changed, there has been a major increase in informal 'having people in' and probably a decline in formal 'entertaining' (JWT, 1981). Clearly the styles of cooking for this have changed too, and daily family eating habits have merged with social habits among younger families. It was expressed well by one person in a group discussion, who said: 'My mum had to cook things that filled us up. People are better off now and we can buy different things. My mum never had a bottle of wine in the house.' The JWT survey showed that 35 per cent of homes stock wine today, and consumption of table wine in the home quadrupled in the 1970s.

Unfortunately there are little hard data about how this has affected the pattern of meals, except for breakfast, which we know has changed substantially over the years, as Table 8 shows.

Consumption studies carried out by Kelloggs since 1972 show that the trend away from cooked breakfast and towards ready-to-eat cereals

Table 8. *How breakfast has changed. From Crawford & Broadley (1938); BMRB menu survey (1972)*

Percent of households serving:	1936/7 (%)	1972 (%)
Eggs	54	32
Bacon	51	20
Porridge	25	13
Ready-to-eat cereals	15	38
Bread/toast	85	72
Tea	95	83
Coffee	8	25

has continued, both for adults and for children. It seems clear that the new individualism has played an important part in this: breakfast is above all the meal in which individual taste can be catered for, individuals can prepare their own and eat it in an informal way, at a time that suits them. Ideas about the role of breakfast have changed too. The tradition of three square meals a day and early to bed, early to rise, has given way to a view of healthy eating less dependent on sheer substance. People still believe in the importance of starting the day with a meal, but its role is seen more as one of balanced refreshment than as one of stoking up for the work of the day ahead.

It may be that the same sort of ideas are beginning to affect other meals, or that people are distinguishing more between 'proper meals' and 'informal meals'. The best data come from the Taylor Nelson Family Food Panel, but only cover five years, which is probably too little to provide more than indications. It seems that lunch is becoming less important and formal, with less substantial food — less meat and potatoes, more eggs and cheese. Tea is moving away from the bread/butter/cake meal towards an evening meal type. The evening meal seems to be becoming more important and substantial. We badly need to be able to relate firmer data on what is actually happening at meals to people's ideas on food and how meals are being planned.

We have even patchier information on the rapidly-changing scene of eating out. The indications are that it is extremely diverse today, and almost certainly has moved from the formal to the informal. Table 9 shows the proportion of women who said they had visited various outlets to eat or drink over the past week. Recent qualitative research is beginning to put together a picture of the ideas and motivations that

Table 9. *Where women eat and drink out.* (*JWT 'Having people in', 1981*)

Per cent of women (aged 16–64) who visited:	In the last month (%)	In the last 7 days (%)
Pub/licensed club	55	33
Self-service cafe/restaurant	23	10
Pub restaurant	16	4
Indian/Chinese restaurant	15	5
McDonalds/Pizza house, etc	14	6
Hotel restaurant	12	4
Steak house	10	2
Other	13	5

lie behind eating out. There appear to be four main types of meal out, two at eating places, two with friends. The only one of them that could be described as formal is the 'proper meal' out: that is planned in advance, the main event of an evening, usually at weekends, people dress up and the meal has the full treatment, with three courses and maybe including steak. Much more common is 'just a meal out': that is much more spontaneous, the meal is incidental to the main purpose of the evening, it tends to be ethnic or fast food, it is quite cheap, happens on weekdays and is particularly a feature of life among young people who move around in groups. There is a similar pattern for eating out at friends' homes, except that formality (the 'dinner party') seems to be very rare indeed. There is the planned meal, which is 'supper', informal and lubricated with wine or beer, part of an evening's entertainment rather than its main purpose, and usually involving a small number of married couples. The fourth type is the spontaneous meal out in someone's home, usually at the end of an evening's entertainment, again involving a few married couples, and almost always based on take-away food. This general picture needs to be quantified, but it is very easy to see how the new patterns of eating out, basically informal, are related to the new individualism.

At the moment this view of changes in eating habits and meal patterns is very impressionistic, and even when there are more data, it will of course not be possible to prove anything. But when I look at what we do know now, it seems to me that the social change hypothesis is much the most convincing. I believe that the most powerful factor affecting the discontinuities in food consumption is the new individualism — the move from formal, respectful, traditional, inherited values to discovered, personal, experimental, informal values.

E. Two disturbing implications

If I am right about the importance of the new individualism, there are disturbing signs that two sorts of people, who both wish to influence eating habits, often run the risk of getting out of touch with the real issues. First, for those who are trying to teach the public about nutrition and healthy eating, there are some doubts about whether they are always going about it in the right way and some awkward questions to answer. For instance, in an era of new individualism and antagonism to the producer bureaucracy, is it realistic to expect people to learn from *institutions*? The hope has often been expressed that people will learn about balanced diets from the examples set in, say, hospitals and schools. But there is certainly evidence from qualitative research of antagonism to school meals (often from those who have no direct experience of them) as dull, stodgy and unattractive. I suspect that the same views are expressed about hospital meals. I am sure this is more a reflection of people's attitudes to the institutions than of the qualities of the food provided. If that is so, no amount of earnest lecturing about how good the diet really is will work. Or one could ask whether the basic approach used in much nutrition education suits the new individualism. Is the approach too analytical? Do teachers teach about nutrients, when what pupils want to know is how to make interesting, exciting, tasty, varied meals as an expression of personal creativity? Does the analytical approach suggest a self-denying and punitive attitude to food? Does it make people feel guilty about liking it? To put it more generally, does some nutrition education start at the wrong end? That is, is it more about what the teacher wants to teach than what the pupil wants to learn? Is nutrition education stuck in the wooden spoon era when most of the pupils have food mixers? Have all the educators understood that unless they start from people's wants and aspirations (whether they approve of them or not), their communications are likely to fail? If any of the criticism implied by these questions is valid, it is not altogether surprising that people become irritated with nutrition 'experts', that they are uninterested in nutritional detail or that they prefer to rely on 'common sense'.

There are equally awkward questions for packaged food manufacturers. They have been under increasing pressures in recent years from the larger retailers, who have massive buying power; from various sorts of official regulators, both from this country and the EEC, who often seem totally out of touch with consumers; and from sheer competition. All too often the result has been an attempt to cheapen processed food: above all, to bring food down to a price. We have seen more and more cheap copies, private label brands and generic brands. The basic awkward question is: can cheapness in food really be what the new individualism is looking for?

There seems to be a marked, and maybe growing, contrast between two different styles of food put before the consumer commercially. On the one hand readers of the popular weekly women's magazines find features showing luscious, stylish, inventive and experimental cooking. In the bolder stores, the variety of interesting delicatessen is growing. The UK is now the main export market for German cheeses, and there are several campaigns under way to interest the British public in foods from continental Europe. On the other hand, generic products are presenting processed food as if it were the same sort of commodity as detergents and kitchen paper. Retailers' advertisements typically stress low price as the main discriminator for their stores, incidentally presenting food as almost anonymous cheap fuel. Manufacturers often appear to believe that the public puts convenience before taste, and produce new products in bland highest-common-factor flavours. Two recently introduced product types — each of which included three brands which featured in lists of the top ten most successful new grocery products — seem to typify the situation: they were instant custard and instant noodles. Both were technically inventive, but both seem light years away from what the new individualists are looking for. If eating habits are really changing, are the food manufacturers keeping up with them?

My conclusion is that eating habits are indeed changing, and that this is the first fundamental change since the end of rationing. I consider that the basic cause is a change in people's attitudes to life and to the food culture, and that it will accelerate. If I am right, there remain these awkward questions both for nutritionists and food manufacturers. But so far most of this is hypothesis. We must hope that the British Nutrition Foundation's research takes us a little nearer to answering the questions.

References

British Market Research Bureau Ltd — BMRB (1972): *The National Menu Survey*. London: BMRB.

BMRB (1978): *Cooking and Recipe Usage in the 1970s*. London: J. Walter Thompson Co. Ltd.

BMRB (1969/70-): *The Target Group Index*. Annual since 1969/70. London: BMRB.

British Nutrition Foundation — BNF (1973): *Food and Nutrition: A Survey of Housewives' Knowledge and Attitudes*. London: British Nutrition Foundation.

BNF (1981): *Eating Behaviour and Attitudes to Food, Nutrition and Health*. Report by S. H. M. King. London: J. Walter Thompson Co. Ltd.

Bourne, R. (1979): The snakes and ladders of the British class system. *New Society*, Feb 8.

Department of Employment (1957-): *Family Expenditure Survey*. Annual since 1957. London: HMSO.

Department of Health and Social Security — DHSS (1979): *Eating for Health*. London: HMSO.

J. Walter Thompson Co. Ltd — JWT (1981): *Having People in: How Women Entertain at Home*. London: J. Walter Thompson Co. Ltd.

Hotels and Catering Economic Development Council (1974-1977): *Trends in Catering: A Study of Eating out*. London: National Economic Development Office.

Kraft Food Ltd (1978): *Survey of Attitudes to Food and Health*. London: Kraft.

McKenzie, J. C. & Mumford, P. (1965): The evaluation of nutrition education programmes. *World Review of Nutrition & Dietetics* 5, pp. 21-31.

Ministry of Agriculture, Fisheries and Food — MAFF (1950-): *Household Food Consumption and Expenditure (National Food Survey)*. Annual since 1950. London: HMSO.

Social Surveys (Gallup Poll) Ltd (1978-): *British Survey of Eating out*. Annual since 1978.

Thomas, J. E. (1979): The relationship between knowledge about food and nutrition and food choice. In *Nutrition and Life-styles*, ed M. R. Turner, pp. 157-167. London: Applied Science Publishers.

Turner, M. R. (editor) (1979): *Nutrition and Life-styles*. London: Applied Science Publishers.

Turner, M. R. (editor) (1981): *Preventive Nutrition and Society*. London: Academic Press.

Turner, M. R. & Gray, J. R. (editors) (1982): *Implementation of Dietary Guidelines*. London: British Nutrition Foundation.

4

'With food convenient for me'
Proverbs 30: 8

DAPHNE GROSE

A. Introduction

We are people. We are tall, short, thin, fat, lazy and workaholics. We make perfect poached eggs *à la bourguignonne*; we cannot boil an egg. We eat porterhouse steaks; we are vegetarians. We are rich, comfortable, poor. We are individuals. We may have habits similar to others who are very like ourselves, but we also have our own peculiar traits. From birth to death others try to influence, mould and change the way we think and the way we behave, and — not least these days — what we eat. Our families, our friends, our teachers, our doctors, influence what we think we should eat and to a lesser extent what we actually eat. The newspapers and magazines we read, and the broadcasts we listen to, in addition to the producers and sellers of food and food-related products, all have a greater or lesser effect on our eating habits. In turn, we as individuals create our own small ripples that may join the ripples from other people's views and actions to produce waves that force changes in social customs and in the marketplace.

B. Individuals in society

1. The individual in the group

The nutritionists and food producers who wish to understand our needs and wishes, or influence our behaviour, cannot begin to study each and every one of us, so they turn to survey research. Producers of food use survey research to obtain indications of what people will buy in the future. This sounds simple, but predicting how individuals will be thinking, feeling, acting in the future is a difficult, complex and uncertain research. Nutritionists, if they are to influence people's thinking about food and their diets, also need an understanding of their knowledge of food, ideas about food, and the reasons why they then act as they do in preparing and eating food. In other chapters of this book the gaps in knowledge about the food people eat at home, outside the home, at meals, between meals, have been made abundantly clear. Equally, the lack of good evidence about the most influential factors which decide the choice, preparation, and presentation of a meal or snack in the home has been demonstrated. Producers and nutritionists undeniably need more survey-based data in order to acquire a greater understanding of people in relation to their food. Yet when this has been obtained I would urge the nutritionists among you to remember that your concern is some 50 million *individuals* and, although practicalities force you to think in terms of groups and sub-groups of people and general trends, if you forget that you are trying to help the individual to make his or her own choice, you will not succeed in influencing people's eating habits. And if you ignore the minority groups you may fail to detect a future trend or a golden opportunity. You may also overlook people who are at risk nutritionally.

Survey research is, in many ways, a far more problematic area than laboratory research. Objective facts — weight, temperature, calorific value or whatever — are straightforward by comparison with the subtlety and the complexity of people's attitudes and opinions, but the producer and nutritionist must venture into precisely this area. If producers of food, or indeed of anything else, are to provide their customers with what they, the customers, want, they must pay attention not only to the 50 per cent, 60 per cent or 70 per cent who are 'very satisfied' but also to the 10 per cent, 5 per cent or 3 per cent who are *not* satisfied and who want something that is not yet, or — perhaps of greater interest — no longer provided. Equally, if the views and habits of the minorities are dismissed as unimportant when attitudinal behaviour survey data is analysed, indications of developing problems or long-term trends may be missed. There is a great temptation to ignore these minorities, but they can be the opinion-formers of tomorrow. There have been a number of examples of small groups of customers resisting the seemingly inevitable changes dictated by the desire for mass markets and finally influencing producer behaviour. The best known example is probably Campaign for Real Ale (CAMRA), but there have been others: who would have dreamed, ten years ago, that a peak time TV commercial break would include an advertisement for wholemeal bread? Yet it happened very recently, and after a debate lasting at least 50 years. (We tend to forget that pre-war the wholemeal versus white bread arguments hit the newspaper headlines.) To the cynic, examples such as these may be a minor delight: to the producer they are, presumably, a source of concern. In fact the food market is beginning to reflect people's increasing interest in health and diet, and in 'fresh' foods. (The long-term decline in the consumption of fresh vegetables may have stabilised, although consumption of fresh green vegetables is particularly low in the younger housewives' families, and fruit consumption continues to rise; when the economy improves growth may take place.) The educationists and scientists should recognise that this may be for them the 'tide in the affairs of men, which taken at the flood, leads on to fortune'. If they can get sound nutritional advice to people at this time, the audience may be very receptive, but, if they fail, people may follow prejudiced guidance from ill-informed sources, and a marvellous opportunity may be lost.

2. The individual influenced by society

There are of course other and older influences on us as individuals. To a greater or lesser extent the individuals' habits are dictated by acceptance or rejection of the customs of the society in which they live, and its past. The eating habits of *Homo sapiens*, from his predecessor's days as a vegetarian in the treetops to the present day American Express card-carrying 'executive' buying exotic foods as status symbols, have been the subject of a number of studies. The evidential trials have apparently become confusing and even faint so that it is difficult to say with any certainty what is man's 'natural' diet. However man is basically omnivorous in nature; a nature which has been modified by local customs and taboos. As a result, each culture has its own strong dietary traditions. This is true of the British Isles. In South-East England, poultry (even if five hundred years ago it might have included tough old swans as well as capons), beef, mutton, ham, bacon, cream, tarts and, of course, bread have appeared in menus down the centuries. Even the poor have had some very small share in this choice. Also, within national cuisines, including the British, there are long-established regional variations. For example, dumplings are an established British filler, but whether they are made with yeast or fat, depends on the county.

Changes do of course take place in eating habits. In this country, these changes have been not only in the basic raw materials of the cuisine, which have been increasing in variety, but in the pattern of meal times, the preparation of the food and the proportion of particular foods eaten. Tea was once taken after dinner. Breakfast, nuncheon, luncheon, brunch have all been midday meals. Dinner, supper, high-tea have been taken at times varying from 3 o'clock in the afternoon to the very late evening. Changes also took place in the character of the meals eaten by aristocratic and, subsequently, middle-class families. For example, the traditional method whereby several courses were placed before the diners at the same time, was replaced in the last century by each course being served consecutively. English literature is full of references to the social nuances of the times meals are eaten and the courses offered. Our society still uses food as a form of signposting within its complex structure, and shows every sign of continuing to do so. The changes, which are social in nature, nonetheless have an effect on people's diets. There is some uncertainty how far the great changes in lifestyle, which have taken place over the last few decades, have modified people's attitudes to what constitutes a proper meal and, more important, changed their habits. Do people think one thing, but behave in a quite different way? Research is taking place, but more is needed if eating habits of the future are to be predicted with any hope of accuracy.

For 400 years, the imperialist ambitions of the Europeans and their travels around the globe brought new foods, particularly the potato, and new ways of preparing foods, to the mother countries. Now the increasingly multi-national and multi-racial nature of almost all societies is leading to the adaptation of one culture's cuisine to extend the range of another cuisine. Immigrants may preserve with devotion in their own homes the niceties of their cuisine, but the people of their adopted countries may select and adapt from that cuisine to suit their own tastes. So the sun probably never sets on the empire of the Italian restauranters, but the subtleties of the pasta change. Recently there was a report in *The Guardian* (29 March, 1982) that pressure from Britain's Muslim and Jewish communities is almost certain to force many of the country's leading food manufacturers to stop using animal fats and other animal extracts in the preparation of many products. These adaptations appear to promise more of variety and choice for us all than the search by scientists for completely new foods. Over time, the diet of individuals will be modified.

Today fashion and current social and political theories continue to modify some people's eating habits. During the last 20 years, among people considered to be nutritionally at risk, have been members of families who have intellectually and emotionally rejected the consumer society and its values. Seeking a new way of life, they have adopted what they consider a more 'natural' diet which has sometimes been so restricted that it has been positively harmful to those with the discipline to follow it. Many more people's diets have been changed by their acceptance of the consumer society and their use of its equipment, its foods and its new lifestyle.

3. The individual and technology

The great changes in the economy and technology in this century have fundamentally changed and improved the diets of the great mass of the people in this country. At the beginning of the century, a large proportion of British people had a monotonous and deficient diet. Ever since the 1930s, there have been great changes. Real wages have increased by about two and a half times. Real disposable income continues to rise (Table 1).

Table 1. *Real personal disposable income per head (Central Statistical Office) Index numbers: 1975 = 100.*

1951	1961	1966	1971	1975	1977	1978	1979
53	74	81	88	100	97	106	111

Most of this additional real disposable income has gone on goods and services and not on food. Overall food consumption has risen since pre-war but bread consumption has about halved.

Households have also changed. Not only have servants long vanished but more and more women, including wives, are working. (In 1980 the percentage of wives working was still over 50 per cent in spite of the effects of recession.)

At the same time technology has added to our choice of food. This year, the New Zealanders are celebrating the centenary since they sent the first frozen lamb to this country. The canning industry is older but appears to have reached a peak in the 1950s and 1960s. Consumption of canned fruit and vegetables has doubled from pre-war. Recently there has been a decline in the consumption of canned fruit, soups and once popular products such as canned milk puddings. In contrast the sale of frozen food is rising steadily. Breakfast cereals (now with bran as well as vitamins) and yogurt are certainly with us for the forseeable future. Milk consumption rose significantly after the 1930s. Now filled milks and semi-skimmed milks are in the shops, although skimmed pasteurised milk is still something of a rarity. This may be a market for development. Less certain is the answer to the question whether young mothers will still be eating 'pot snacks' in five years or alternatively whether by then that portion of the population who at this time have never tried one will have been hooked. Or will the increasing interest of many people in 'simpler' foods direct the food industry to 'fresh' foods ready prepared for use. Certainly, the new controlled atmosphere methods in storage and packaging should increase the keeping qualities of these foods.

While food technology has advanced, so too has the domestic appliance industry. Today the main room in a house may well be the modern kitchen. The colour magazines are full of advertisements for them. One such advertisement says there are 4500 different units to choose from. Such kitchens with their range of ovens, hobs and grills, micro-wave ovens, extractor hoods, fridges, freezers, dishwashers, food mixers, food processors (sending us back to the liquid foods of infancy), pasta machines and so on and so on may cost many thousands of pounds. Most people make do with a self-assembly collection of units and a somewhat small range of equipment. Ownership of some appliances is shown in Table 2.

Table 2. *Ownership of household appliances (Central Statistical Office)*

| | percentage of British households | | | | |
	1961	1970	1975	1979	1980
Refrigerators	25	63	84	92	93
Freezers	—	—	13	25	28
Fridge-freezers	—	—	—	15	19
Food and drink mixers	5	24	40	47	50

The market for refrigerators has now reached saturation point. Increased sales of small refrigerators suggest that there may be households buying second refrigerators for rooms other than the kitchen, while on the replacement market, fridge/freezers are leading the market. Not surprisingly all this chill equipment in the home is having an effect on food consumption. The National Food Survey shows that freezer owners eat more poultry and carcase meat per person per week than non-owners. (The difference does not seem to relate to income alone.) In addition Birds Eye estimates that by 1984 freezer owners will be responsible for about 70 per cent of the value of frozen food sales in Britain. The freezer is also receiving an increasingly wide variety of foods, for example there is a rising sale of frozen sausages. At the same time, people are growing more vegetables. In the late 1950s home grown vegetables contributed about 15 per cent of all fresh vegetables which were then being eaten. A decline then set in which was arrested by the recession of the 1970s and home grown vegetable production is now higher than in the late 1950s (Mintel, 1982). Some of these vegetables are frozen at home. In fact some freezer owners freeze anything they can lay their hands on — suitable or unsuitable. Some produce is blanched and some is not. Arguably the freezer will in time be shown to have been a more important influence on our eating habits than anything else.

4. Enjoying food

Sometimes I detect a note of regret, or even disapproval, among food producers that people no longer spend (as they did until the end of the 1950s) a third of their total expenditure on food. (Working class households in 1937–38 were spending nearly half of their total expenditure on food). In 1980, expenditure on food was about 20 per cent of total expenditure, with about 8 per cent spent on alcohol and tobacco, and over 10 per cent on the owning and running of a motor car (British Labour Statistics, 1971; Family Expenditure Survey, 1980). For the majority of us, food is not just a matter of 'daily bread', but of pleasure and enjoyment. Once the family was held together by Sunday lunch, today it may be equally well held together by a trip in the family car to the seaside. The livestock farmer may find it hard to accept that he has to compete with the petrol company, but that is the reality. The General Household Survey classifies 'going out for a meal or a drink' as a leisure activity. This dichotomy of food as a necessity for life and as a pleasurable activity, bedevils so much of our response to the advice we receive on our diets. Nutritionists need to find the obverse to the 'It's naughty but it's nice' advertising slogan.

 ## 5. Eating out

Unfortunately, the National Food Survey relates mainly to food purchased for consumption in the home. Yet 16 per cent of all expenditure on food falls outside this category and the only section of the food business showing growth is the 'eating out' section. For some people, a large number of their meals and snacks are eaten away from home, and so the balance of their diet is decided by the nature of the food provided in catering establishments. A study of this food might reveal a need to revise the figures now accepted as reasonable estimates of actual nutrient intake. The 1982 Gallup Menu Survey for the *Caterer and Hotelkeeper*, based on responses from caterers, showed that the new forms of fast food and take-aways have now moved into all parts of the country. The survey also suggests that the majority of us prefer to eat fairly lightly and informally at lunchtime. (How many beers are drunk, sausages and packets of crisps are eaten at midday? Or is it now wine and quiche?) Now for more formal eating out, prawn cocktail, steak, chips and peas, and cheesecake remains the most popular type of meal.

Between meals eating is changing, more savoury (salty?) snacks and less sweets being consumed.

6. Alcohol

The general level of alcohol consumption has risen consistently since the end of the second world war. According to the Office of Health Economics (1981) Britain entered the post-war period of the 1950s 'as "sober" a country as it has ever been in its recorded history'. Since then there has been a return to higher drinking levels. Recently there has been a levelling off but this may be due to the recession. Whilst beer remains far and away the most popular form of alcohol, accounting for approximately two-thirds of all alcohol consumption, wine sales are now four times the 1900 level and are continuing to rise rapidly. Alcohol is a significant part of some people's energy intake.

7. The individual

The influence of society is obviously important, but again I must stress our individuality. No one person is like any other person. We are born with our own individual physical and psychological peculiarities. Why, for example, do some people find red foods repulsive? Why do others for example find milk or a boiled egg repugnant? Why do some children, without encouragement from their parents, become vegetarians? How to explain the man who last year was taken into hospital suffering from the effects of a diet of kippers in jam, eels in lemon curd and sheep's eyes in custard? (He began the diet to raise money for charity and grew to like it!) Easier to understand is the ascetic's small regard for food and the unhappy person's use of it for solace. Even within families, there will be marked differences in food preferences and the amount eaten. There is too, of course, the accepted fact that our individual need for energy and nutrients vary. This variety presents a challenge to those who would change what we eat.

I think Professor J. C. McKenzie was right when he wrote that if food consumption patterns change they usually change because individuals want them to (McKenzie, 1981). Rising and unacceptable prices will reduce consumption, as will shortages, but, otherwise, change comes because groups of people see a food as having a new status or place in society, or having some new value for themselves personally, so they start eating it, or, conversely, because they think a food will harm them or they become bored with it, they stop eating it. (Boredom, I am convinced, is the main hazard for the food processor who produces for the mass market.) There are indications at this time that habits are changing. Many people have for some time been more aware that there is such a thing as positively protecting one's health and that a healthy person is usually more attractive than an unhealthy one. The idea that diet and health are linked has been spreading through society. (Penguin Books are said to have sold nearly a million copies of Audrey Eyton's low calorie:high fibre diet book, *The F-Plan*, between May and July 1982.) Of course there are still many, many individuals who say: To hell with it all. But there are enough individuals who do care for it to be vital that they should be helped to translate their concern into sound action.

C. The multiplicity of messages

1. The nutritionists' messages

Today, each of us is receiving a multiplicity of messages from those who would influence our eating habits. Many of us are naïve enough to think that science deals in absolutes and certainties, so we are particularly confused by the nutritionists' changes of view. If you have been brought up to believe in the health giving properties of spinach, liver and milk, it is difficult to modify one's ideas and accept that benefits and disadvantages may be combined in one natural product. So, already somewhat bewildered, we are further confused by the public disagreements of the experts. The public battles of competing schools of thought create a noise which may drown out any intelligible message we might otherwise receive, and the commercial persuaders add to the confusion.

2. The suppliers of dietary supplements

'Healthy' eating is undoubtedly fashionable. Some people's fear that their own diet may be deficient is a temptation for those promoting dietary supplements. In May of this year, I scanned *Good House-keeping*: one advertisement for dietary supplements offered me 'The new balanced way to positive health' with several products including 'Natural balance multi-vitamins enriched with alfalfa'. The small print says of the products '. . . helps to counterbalance what is wrong with the way we eat today. Alfalfa, with such a wealth of nutrients that it has been called the Father of all Foods . . .'. Another advertisement read 'If you have a properly balanced diet, you should be getting all the vitamins you need — including vitamin E. Food such as wholewheat bread, eggs, cereals, sesame seeds and cod liver oil are all rich in vitamin E. Even so, you would have to eat a great deal of all of them to get as much vitamin E as just one vitamin E tablet can provide'. (How much vitamin E do I need, I ask myself?) Yet a third advertisement talks about '. . . a unique combination of all the B vitamins plus vitamin C, which many years' research has shown to provide an ideal balance of those vitamins the body requires when under physical strain'. Each advertisement made the regulatory nod to a balanced diet, but the message for me was clear: I was unlikely to be getting a balanced and healthy diet which would be sufficient for my personal needs, and I was being invited to increase the £20 million spent last year on vitamin pills.

Some promotional messages suggest that it is very difficult to achieve a well-balanced diet. An advertisement in the July (1982) issue of *Family Circle* says '. . . But even a well-balanced diet may not be enough. It's a fact that vitamins and minerals are easily destroyed or lost by the prolonged cooking, storage and over-processing of food. So if you're not careful about what you eat and the life you lead, you may well risk suffering from a deficiency.' The leaflet in the packs of a multi-vitamin brand leader states: 'Modern methods of preserving food, over-cooking, freezing and long-term storage of food can destroy many of the vitamins'. The same leaflet says lack of a vitamin can cause serious problems, for example, lack of vitamin A can cause night blindness, vitamin B neuritis, vitamin C scurvy. Among those who are listed as being likely to need supplementary vitamins are people who regularly eat out including business executives and working men and women who take their midday meal in a restaurant, cafe or canteen. Bombarded by this message, all ages and social classes are buying supplements. Given that some individuals believe that more must be better, may there not be risks in this encouragement of uncritical swallowing of vitamins and minerals? Should a strong counter-message be published? Should the advertisers be required to be more restrained?

3. What messages are people hearing?

Faced with the disputes about fat and heart disease, and the difficulty of deciding if one's own diet is balanced and adequate, there are times when I, and I am sure many others, think to ourselves: a curse on all your houses. In spite of this, some of the nutritionists' messages are getting through. J. C. McKenzie (1979) found that respondents (505) asked to identify which of the health problems they had previously indicated as being of importance were influenced by food consumption, named overweight (54 per cent), heart trouble (47 per cent), and high blood pressure (28 per cent). A third of respondents in the 1981 Health Education Council survey said improving the diet was a method of preventing heart disease.

The Consumers' Association in 1981 undertook some limited research to help us in our thinking on terms used in relation to slimming claims. Four group discussions were held amongst a sample of 35 women living in the Greater London area. The participants were balanced as to age and socio-economic classification. The sample was recruited on the basis of half being slimmers and half being non-slimmers. During the discussions led by a trained psychologist, however, we obtained an impression that this distinction was in-appropriate. Many women today may either constantly watch their weight, or that of a family member, without describing themselves as 'slimming' or 'being on a diet'. There was no doubt in the minds of respondents that the majority of women today are aware that the only way to lose weight, or to maintain a stable weight, is to control total food intake. If this is true, a simple but important message has been successfully transmitted. McKenzie (1979) suggested that it is women who are more aware of the dangers of overweight so fashion too may have played its part.

Individual respondent's comments made during the Consumers' Association discussion groups were interesting:

'I think I buy things now more for a balanced diet than for slimming reasons. I notice more if there is protein, vegetable and that sort of thing — and we eat bread now for the roughage'

'It's nutrition now, not dieting'

'We don't eat fattening foods now out of habit. Low cholesterol diets are for health. It's not that it's low fattening — I know that — as eggs are good for a diet but not for cholesterol'

'Bread and potatoes are now good for you as they are low in fat'.

There are a number of points to be noted. 'Diet' has a double meaning. There is almost certainly some misunderstanding about the nature and importance of cholesterol. The message about fat has become confused. Some of those in the discussion groups associated 'low fat' with 'low cholesterol' and assumed that foods marked 'low fat' meant 'high in polyunsaturated fat'. There were a few who were clear what each term meant, but many admitted that they were very confused about it all. 'High in polyunsaturated fats' seemed like a double negative. 'Low calorie' and 'low fat' were perceived as being good, and something 'high' in a substance ought to be bad. Even some of the basic knowledge is still missing. Some thought that calories were present only, or mainly, in sugars, starches or fat.

Some myths may not be easy to dislodge. The Department of Agricultural Marketing of Newcastle upon Tyne has found in its consumer attitude research that different types of meat are considered to have varying values from a nutritional point of view. This is interesting, because these views appear to have only a limited effect on what people buy. Over the last 25 years, meat consumption overall has shown little variation, but there have been quite significant changes in the consumption of different types of meat from time to time. Beef is particularly sensitive to overall levels of income. It is the first of the meats to suffer when incomes in real terms decline. However, it retains a special place in people's affections — as stated by a spokesman for the Meat Promotion Executive (1980) at a conference: '. . . beef is very special in that many consumers believe that it has a series of benefits that cannot be provided by any other food, that these benefits are central to a healthy family's diet. These beliefs do not rest on rational claims — they are strongly emotionally held, and it is vitally important that we accept them and use them in our advertising'. Beef is part of the national heritage, so it must have special properties. Such views and gut reactions are not easily countered and possibly we need a few such myths in our lives. We must remember, however, that they exist, and be sure that they are not fostered to the point that they really have an undue influence on what we do and do not eat.

4. What information do we want?

Some of us may not want any information about the balance of food needed for a healthy diet. Others may actually wish for and even need, for therapeutic purposes, detailed data about specific foods. Each of us who wants information will also want it in a form that is easily understood and usable and relevant to us as individuals. As individuals, we have to be able to apply the information to our own needs, which will vary according to our age, our work, our build, our health, our general metabolism, our preferences, our appetite, and our lifestyle. Most of us do not want precise scientific data because, however intelligent we may be, we do not have the time or inclination to master such material. We are not interested in nutrients, but the amount of shepherds pie we can eat if our diet is to remain balanced. The majority of us are not willing to change fundamentally our customary methods of cooking and the pattern of our eating; Jackie Craske (1982) has recently demonstrated this.

5. How difficult is it to follow a nutritionist's message?

One of the most commonly heard messages today is the need to reduce fat consumption. This may seem one of the simpler pieces of nutritional advice for people to follow. We are told potatoes and fish are good for us. But I am sure that I am not alone in liking them together in a pie with lashings of cheese sauce and fluffy creamed potatoes and with smoked fish and shell fish included. These are 'acceptable' foods turned into a dish full of calories and fat. Yet food has always been for pleasure as well as sustenance. We need guidance on how we can fit our gastronomic pleasures into a diet which will not be harmful. In addition, we need help in assessing all those foods we eat out of the home and the convenience foods we buy from the supermarket. We may even need help with traditional 'fresh' foods. In a recent survey on minced meat, the Consumers' Association obtained indications that people's perception of the percentage of fat in mince bought was less than the fat found on analysis. Certainly, it is difficult to assess the hidden fat in compound products.

There are, of course, medical and other experts who do not think the advice to reduce fat is sufficient and that more precise guidance on particular fats should be given. In January this year, the Consumers' Association (1982) published an article on food and health: heart disease, which examined, in particular, the relationship between dietary fat and heart disease, and which went on to recommend that people should aim to reduce their total fat consumption and worry less about animal vs vegetable or saturated vs polyunsaturated. The article caused something of a furore and we have been attacked from all sides although we did have support from the British Nutrition Foundation. We stand firmly by what we have said, however, on the grounds that our aim was to give practical, sensible advice which could easily be followed by the vast majority of ordinary people. It is clear that it is very difficult to summarise adequately the wealth of evidence on a subject as complicated as this. It is equally clear that there are real problems in presenting a summary view simply, clearly and concisely, in such a way that misunderstandings will not arise. What matters at the end of the day is that sound, practical advice should be given to people. The scientific and medical evidence as collected and evaluated by the expert committees, which are comprised essentially of scientists, medics or other academics, may lead to a conclusion that in an ideal world people should replace one fat with another, but it seems to us that this is not practical advice. In the main, people do not know what sort of fats they are eating now, so how can they sensibly change from one to another. The first step ought to be to reduce total fat consumption — and we gave advice about how to do this. Other changes could be recommended later, but fundamental changes in dietary habits cannot be expected to happen overnight.

6. Does product advertising help or hinder?

Product advertising has very great limitations as a source of information. The message, even if not biased in favour of the product, is inevitably over-simplified. For example the current All-bran advertisement says: 'Fibre absorbs and holds water, speeding up the elimination of waste. This action helps prevent constipation, piles and gallstones. And, according to recent research, it may help prevent bowel cancer and heart disease, too'. Do people fully appreciate the qualifications of the last sentence? At which moment in the development of a diet and health hypothesis is it wise to make such claims? For example, the Food Standards Committee refused in 1980 to propose appropriate labelling rules for fibre because of the absence of any agreed definition of dietary fibre and the current state of nutritional understanding. Unfortunately this leaves the way open for labellers each to do their own thing. In addition, if dietary advice becomes too closely associated in people's minds with one product and brand, they may fail to absorb the full message, in this case the place of dietary fibre in the diet. (I know that in the case of All-bran, Kelloggs offer, as a give-away for two coupons from their packs, a fibre chart, but in terms which leaves the original message intact.) The legislators have decided to ban therapeutic claims for foods. The Food Labelling Regulations 1980, which are due to come into effect next in January 1983, ban claims that a food is capable of preventing, treating or curing human disease, either expressly or by implication, in labelling or advertising, unless the food has a product licence under the Medicines Act.

The battles between the margarine and butter industries have clearly demonstrated another problem. The British Code of Advertising Practice prohibits direct claims for polyunsaturated fats. To be really effective this sound piece of control ought to have been supported by the labelling of margarines to indicate the saturated and poly-unsaturated fat content. As it was, many people picked up the distorted message that all soft margarines were 'healthy'. Last year the Butter Information Council struck back with a campaign against margarine. Commenting on this campaign the Code of Advertising Practice Committee wrote: 'where complicated medical or scientific issues were the subject of advertisements addressed to the public, the advertiser was under a particular obligation to present the subject matter in such a way as to avoid the possibility of lay readers being led to a false appreciation of the situation. In particular, the way in which the case was put overlooked the very substantial degree of agreement between the experts as to the general desirability of the reduction of the intake of all kinds of fats in the diet'. This comment clearly indicates the impracticality of expecting advertisers to offer truly sound nutritional advice. This in turn must raise the question of other forms of promotion such as public relations, press releases, sponsored seminars and other ways of associating one product with good health. If there is going to be an increasing number of research discoveries associating particular foods or nutrients with therapeutic properties and pathological conditions, then, if the public are not to become a mixture of neurotic food faddists and eat, drink and be merry don't carers, the academic world must exercise care in presenting the results of research and the food trade must show restraint in exploiting such material. This is an area in which the food trade might well regulate itself. Last year (1981), Tim Fortescue of the Food and Drinks Industry Council discussed and commented on the harm which can be done when organisations, whose chief object is to promote one commodity, defend their commodity against any attack by a nutritional or other scientist by a counter-attack by another expert. I agree. People become confused and the reputation of the food trade as a whole suffers. However, the remedy is in the trade's hands.

7. Food labelling

Do people want processed foods to be labelled with their nutrient contents? Carbohydrate and calorie values would be some guide for weight-watchers following particular dietary regimes, but would they help most of us to devise balanced family diets? Fat declaration would certainly help if reduction in fat intake is an aim of national nutritional policy but this does not necessarily help an individual devise a diet providing a balance of essential nutrients. The pressure for nutrient labelling both here and overseas has come from doctors, scientists and nutritionists and not so much the consumer organisations. We are convinced that there needs to be more research about methods of giving nutritional and nutrient information to people so that they can understand it and use it, and in a format that will not discourage them so they think the data are too complex for them to try and use. In addition, we think it is imperative that if nutritional labelling is going to be given on more foods that, at the same time, information should also be provided on the fresh foods. The listing of nutrients in processed foods could only mislead people into thinking they are of greater food value than fresh foods. Nevertheless we recognise, and I must add, appreciate, the initiatives taken by some firms in providing nutritional information on their products. They are, however, using different criteria for deciding for example the servings on which the nutrient data are based. There is a need for some simple guidelines on voluntary nutritional labelling since it seems certain that the government does not intend to act on the recommendations of the Food Standards Committee's *Second Report on Claims and Misleading Descriptions* (1980).

8. *A balanced diet*

The more interest I have taken in food and nutrition, the clearer it has become to me that most people want and need simple guidelines for achieving a balanced diet. Some, of course, want much more and they have the right to have it in some form, but for most the information has to be simple. Before providing this information, however, the experts must decide what they mean by a balanced diet.

In a speech earlier this year, Mrs Peggy Fenner, Parliamentary Secretary at the Ministry of Agriculture, Fisheries, and Food said: 'I accept that a well-balanced diet is necessary for good health. But how do you define a well-balanced diet? I am quite sure that if that question was directed to a group of nutritionists, there would be considerable variations in the advice which they offered.' I hope the British Nutrition Foundation is clear what it means. Next, there is a need to discover what different people think the term 'balanced diet' means, so that the guidelines can be written with an appreciation of people's conception and misconception of the subject. Nor, I suggest, is it enough to base the advice on the basic food groups alone without guidance on the way the foods are prepared and cooked, and the quantities to be eaten. In all cases meals, snacks and food on the plate must be the starting point for the advice if individuals are to be able to relate it to themselves and their lifestyles. Finally, one leaflet, one booklet, suitable for all of us will not be possible. Information needs to be aimed at particular groups with different ideas or eating habits. Each of us needs to be able to relate the message to ourselves personally.

9. The beliefs around us

All of us, from our childhood onwards, are constantly benefiting from the wisdom and knowledge, and also being misled by the false ideas and views, of those with whom we come into contact. The chemistry teacher who thinks all processed foods are junk and full of nasty chemicals may pass this view to the child who tells its mother, confirming her own ideas, gleaned from half hearing a radio programme. This is the way ideas spread in society. All educationists, and all those in a position to influence opinion, are therefore important to the nutritionist. At the 1980 BNF Annual Conference, Tony Smith of the British Medical Journal explored in his paper the subject of the media (Smith, 1981). The problems in persuading an audience not to see everything as either absolutely black or pure white, and to accept the need for qualification, are not likely to be overcome easily. However, advice given frequently with complete conviction and confidence, and which the people who hear it find sensible and can relate to, will in the end take root and flourish.

The food industries have a part to play in helping to create an informed and sceptical public who will question things, but not be misled by, for example, anti-technology prejudices. Many processed foods have a high nutritional value. Other processed foods are largely fun foods and have a low calorific value or a high calorific value, but mainly from sugars. Independent bodies, such as the British Nutrition Foundation and my own organisation, can help people to distinguish between these types of food, and to appreciate the particular characteristics of each group of products. The food industry can help in another way. Food technology is moving further and further away from original craft or kitchen cooking. Even 'fresh' foods are now treated to lengthen storage life. People are largely unaware of these developments, and the industry in general thinks that this ignorance is best for everyone. The industry fears that if people knew how foods were processed they would refuse to buy the products. This is unwise. In the end, the facts come out and then people think they have been deceived, and therefore suspect the value of the foods. The industry would be wise to explain to its customers new technologies and give the facts about the nutritional value of foods treated in specific ways. At the same time, the industry's technologists would be wise to take account of current consensus views on nutritional issues, although I do not think it is the job of the industry to tell us what we should eat.

D. Conclusions

The messages we are now receiving about the ways to achieve a healthy diet are confused and confusing. Even if the message was strong and clear we would be likely to adapt it to our own natural inclinations and our personal circumstances, but when we receive conflicting recommendations, selection of the message we would prefer to hear and find personally most convenient comes naturally and easily. This could be bad for us. Then we may misunderstand the message. Add to this that some of the recommendations are not practicable, or at least difficult to follow, and we may well decide to curse all nutritionists and others who try to tell us what is and is not good for us to eat. Even if we try to follow what we think is the advice being given to us, our knowledge or perception of the foods we buy may be false. So we need help, but help based on a sound understanding of our knowledge, ideas, attitudes and way of life.

The *New English Bible* translates the title I have chosen as 'provide me only with the food I need'. Few of us could by choice live with such discipline, but equally many of us would like to know just what we do need. Tell us what we need and give us the information in a way that permits us to use it as is convenient to each of us as an individual. Above all, don't try to stop us enjoying our food.

References
(*Denotes general reference)

Central Statistical Office (1980): *Social Trends No. 10*. London: HMSO.*
Central Statistical Office (1981): *Social Trends No. 11*. London: HMSO.*
Central Statistical Office (1982): *Social Trends No. 12*. London: HMSO.*
Cleminson, James (1982): How will food businesses evolve? *Chemistry and Industry* 9, 287–292.*
Consumers' Association (1982): Food and health: heart disease. *Which?* January 1982, 10–12.
Craske, J. (1982): Dietary change. *Home Economics*, June 1982, 7–8.

Department of Employment (1971): *British Labour Statistics. Historical Abstract 1886-1968*. London: HMSO.

Department of Employment (1980): *Family Expenditure Survey 1980*. London: HMSO.

Ebling, J. (1982): Man the consumer. *Chemistry and Industry* 10, 315-321.*

Economist Intelligence Unit (1982): *Retail Business* 287-289. London: Economist.*

Food Standards Committee (1980): *Second Report on Claims and Misleading Descriptions*. London: HMSO.

Fortescue, T. V. N. (1981): The role of the food manufacturing industry in nutrition education. In *Preventive Nutrition and Society*, ed M. R. Turner. London: Academic Press.

Gallup Menu Survey (1982): *Hotel and Caterer*, 15 April.

Johnston, J. P. (1977): *A Hundred Years Eating*. Dublin: Gill and MacMillan.

McKenzie, J. (1979): The consumers' view of problems and priorities in nutrition. *The Proceedings of Nutrition Society* 38, 219-223.

McKenzie, J. (1981): Evolution of eating habits in countries of the European Community. In *Symposium on Nutrition, Food Technology and Nutritional Information*, London, 19-20 March 1980. (Commission of the European Communities, Eur 7085 EN, Brussels and Luxembourg).

Meat Promotion Executive (1980): *Proceedings of National Conference on Beef Production and Marketing, 2-3 December 1980* (jointly sponsored by Elanco Products and Livestock Farming).

Mintel (1982): *Market Intelligence Reports*, January 1982, 15.

National Food Survey (Annual Report): *Household Food Consumption and Expenditure*. London: HMSO.*

Office of Health Economics (1981): *Alcohol — Reducing the Harm*. (Office of Health Economics, London).

Richardson, D. P. (1982): Changing public ideas about the wholesomeness of food. *Nutrition Bulletin* 1, 31-38.*

Simoons, F. J. (1976): Food habits as influenced by human culture: approaches in anthropology and geography. In *Report of the Dahlem Workshop on appetite and food intake*, ed T. Silverstone. Life Sciences Research Report 2. Berlin: Abakon.*

Smith, A. J. (1981): Nutrition and the media. In *Preventive Nutrition and Society*, ed M. R. Turner. London and New York: Academic Press.

5

The manufacturer's response to changing consumer preference

HOWARD PHILLIPS

A. Introduction

The changes which have taken place in our living environment, our society, and our way of thinking since the 1950s have been profound, and have been instrumental in the formation of a generation of people who are now the vitally important consumers of manufactured food products.

The characteristics of tomorrow's consumer will similarly be formed by a further complex and independent set of factors; some of these are identifiable now, some are easily predicted, but some are beyond explicit analytical assessment and can only be anticipated (if at all) by more intuitive means.

This chapter deals with some recent changes in society that have formed the characteristics of today's consumers, illustrating, wherever possible, how food manufacturers, and particularly my company, have responded to these changes. I shall concentrate on frozen food, which is an important part of my company's business — but the examples are more than valid because it is quite clear that the growth of frozen food is linked to a number of the key changes in consumer preferences over the last 10 years. I shall attempt to project how all or some of the existing characteristics of today's consumer may or may not change during the rest of this decade.

B. Structure of society

Firstly, let us look at how the actual structure of our society has changed in recent years. Fewer children are being born and this has quite naturally resulted in very little growth in the population. For the food manufacturer this, in effect, means that we have a static total market, or what is sometimes described as the 'constant stomach'. In other words, manufacturers' growth for one particular food product must necessarily come at the expense of a decline in another food product. The food manufacturer's challenge, therefore, is to identify areas of growth to compensate for any products in their (or their competitors') portfolios that are in danger of obsolescence.

Over 50 per cent of all married women now work and this has produced fundamental changes in requirements for food. For a start, the working housewife no longer has the time or the inclination to cook after a day at work away from the home; she is, therefore, much more receptive to products she can prepare quickly and conveniently, that provide her with value for money and which are readily accepted by the members of her family. There are numerous examples of products which have shown strong growth (increased sales) as a result of this trend. To name a few, there are the prepared meat products such as our own 'Grillsteaks' product, prepared fish dishes such as 'Fish in sauce' and 'Cod in batter', and even the ultimate in convenience, the 'Oven chip', which requires no peeling and no deep fat frying, just 20 minutes in the oven.

There has been a significant growth in the number of one and two person households as a result of the higher divorce rate, an increase in the elderly population, young people are leaving home earlier and there is an increase in households with no dependent children. In 1961 the average British household contained just over three people, households with no dependent children represented 56 per cent of the total and single person households accounted for 12 per cent of the total.

In stark contrast, by 1981 the average household size was 2.68 people and households with no dependent children had risen to 63 per cent of the total — a direct result of an increase in the number of childless couples and a compression of the child-bearing period.

Single-person households in 1981 had risen to nearly one-quarter of the population. 'Mr & Mrs Average', portrayed by the media and the Chancellor of the Exchequer at Budget time, as a working man with two children and a housewife represents, in fact, only 5 per cent of all households. The impact of changes in household structures has been profound and extensive. This, in turn, has undermined the economics of many traditional home-based activities, such as the preparation of family meals, and has increased the demand for convenient, single-serving portions of various foods and drinks.

As you would expect, these three factors have greatly influenced the growth of frozen food over the last decade. Frozen foods represent total convenience by their very nature — no mess, no fuss, little preparation. Frozen foods come in all shapes and sizes, individual portions for single-person households right up to large packs for the working housewife with three children who no longer has the time to shop every day, or even every week. Frozen foods also provide excellent value for money and this method of food processing preserves all the inherent qualities of food without significantly affecting its natural qualities.

C. Influence of technology

Running parallel with these changes in household structure have been the influences of technology. As man's scientific knowledge has progressed, so his ability to develop new products for the home has increased at a rapid pace; indeed a recent analysis indicated that the home has become virtually a centre for work, leisure and entertainment, with many items considered as essential by the householder of today which would not have been dreamed of by those living in 1950 — just over 30 years ago.

Technology in the home tends to fall into two basic categories: items which are for convenience and items which provide entertainment. Among those items which are for convenience, there is, as you would expect, a high concentration of items that are designed to save time in the kitchen, again emphasising the trend away from traditional cooking methods.

One development, particularly close to our own heart, which has had a huge impact on food consumption patterns, has been the freezer. Ownership has soared from 3 per cent of households in 1970 to 57 per cent last year, and this growth has been almost entirely due to the continuing consumer demand for convenience. With a freezer the housewife can save money, and she can make the sort of spontaneous menu decisions that would not be possible without the advent of the modern larder — the freezer. Ross Foods was, in fact, one of the first major frozen food companies to recognise this trend by introducing a range of home freezer products in large packs during the 1970s, aimed specifically at the blossoming freezer centre market. It is interesting to note that even today the trend in the market is clearly towards larger packs. There has been in recent years, however, a trend towards medium-sized packs as the size of freezer units has tended to be reduced.

Another area of growth has been in the sales of kitchen appliances such as food mixers and blenders, penetration having increased from

5 per cent to 50 per cent in the last 20 years, and again it is convenience which has influenced sales. The microwave oven is another convenience tool which is beginning to make its mark. Penetration is only about 1 per cent of households at present, but there are signs that the microwave will become yet another weapon in the householder's convenience armoury during the 1980s. By 1990 penetration is projected to increase to 8 per cent of households, and as a food manufacturer we are currently monitoring very closely this development with a view to providing microwave cooking instructions and microwaveable food packaging, as well as developing products specifically for microwave cooking.

The list of convenience kitchen equipment is endless, growing all the time with items such as sandwich toasters, slow-cooking pots and food processors, all gaining steadily in popularity. Again it is extremely important for the food manufacturer to remain aware of these trends and to develop products that are compatible with these constantly changing consumer habits.

On the other side of the coin is the blossoming home entertainments industry. There are few homes today without a television set; some recent research shows that viewing hours per household have increased from 4.7 hours per day in 1971 to 5.1 hours per day in 1980.

This must have impact on our way of life, focusing family attention away from the more traditional evening pursuits and almost requiring a completely new meal-eating regimen, geared to speed, convenience and the ability to be balanced on the knee! But television is only the start of a whole new age of home entertainments, of which television games, home computers and video recorders are just the tip of the iceberg.

D. Changing social attitudes

While the influences of technology and broad social changes can be relatively easily identified, there are also some less tangible changes in our social attitudes which should be considered, but which are much more difficult to correlate with changes in buying habits as far as the food manufacturer is concerned.

1. Role sharing

The blurring of the roles of the male and the female means that both men and women are now involved in such activities as housework and, importantly from the manufacturers' standpoint, shopping and cooking.

2. New values

Today's consumer is much more concerned about personal creativity and job satisfaction, intellectual and spiritual development and physical fitness. They tend to prefer natural foods and natural fabrics, and generally, being better educated, they are now much more concerned about ingredients and health elements of the food that they eat. They are more interested in quality than appearance, and 'routine' is more often rejected in favour of 'spontaneity'.

3. Lifestyles

Today's consumers tend to have many more varied interests such as foreign food, cooking, further education, the performing arts, reading and music. Their informal life-style leads them to use more and more good quality convenience foods, take-home foods and snacks where necessary.

For the food industry, these changes in social attitude and structure have had a considerable impact. More people are prepared to eat on the move than ever before and there is greater concern about the goodness of the food that we eat. There is an increasing demand for more variety in our diet than ever before.

E. The shopping basket of today

If we relate these changes in social attitude to the actual food purchases, we find that a number of significant changes have occurred in the shopping basket of today compared to 10 or 15 years ago. For instance, there is a greater variety of foods available. Again I shall use examples from my own company to illustrate the points I am going to make. The current Ross Retail and Home Freezer product list alone includes over 150 different products, plus numerous alternative choices within specific food sectors. For instance, there are three varieties of fish finger including 'Cod supervalue' and our recently introduced 'Jumbo cod finger'. There are four choices of Peas — 'Garden', 'Petit pois', 'Economy' and 'Aylesbury minted'. There are also various types of 'Burgers' designed to meet the needs of the housewife who is serving high tea to her children, and of the housewife who is serving a main evening meal for her husband, where she has the option of serving a quarterpounder 'Burger' or our recently introduced 'Grillsteak' product, which provides all the benefits of convenience frozen meat, but in a more substantial and satisfying format.

There are more foreign foods eaten today. Ever since people started travelling abroad and developing tastes for new foods, the food industry has sought to meet demands by introducing ranges of exotic dishes. I should mention that this trend has also been supplemented by the influx of a whole range of cosmopolitan restaurants introducing the English palate to such things as Chinese, Indian, and Italian food. Again, to use the Ross product list as an example, we as a company offer a whole range of products of foreign derivation, ranging from individual curries and pizzas for the retail market, to multi-portion entrées, such as, 'Chicken Spanish style', 'Chilli con carne' and 'Lasagne' for the catering/fast food market.

As I have already mentioned, there is much more emphasis today on convenience food. A good example of this is the choice now available in the humble potato product. Two years ago potato products meant chips; today there is an ever growing selection of potato products ranging from 'Bubble and squeak', 'Oven crunches' (specifically designed to cook in the oven) to 'Potato noisettes' and 'Jacket scollops', which can be grilled, fried or even oven cooked, and incidentally some having the added benefit, from a nutritional standpoint, of having their skins left on.

There is much more concern today about the goodness of the food that we eat. The whole area of health, dieting, slimming and concern about substances conceived as harmful, has potentially major implications for the food manufacturer. There has been a shift away from negative concern, ie avoiding foods which are bad, towards a positive approach of concern with the food and activities which tend to promote good health. From our own standpoint at Ross, ample evidence can be found of our response to this trend in the development of products like our 100 per cent 'Beefburgers', our 100 per cent beef 'Grillsteak' product, which I mentioned earlier, and our recently introduced 'Wholemeal base pizza', all of which have been introduced in the last two years.

There are many more packaged commodities today. For example, you can now buy a great many products in packs which is obviously much more convenient and much more hygienic, if less quaint, than the old fashioned way of buying products loose. Vegetables are perhaps the most obvious examples, but you could also include frozen filleted fish, which we market under the Ross Fish Shop range, and even frozen pastry.

There are also many more varieties of pack sizes available to the shopper in the supermarket today, catering for the needs of the single person household, the two-person household, right up to the much larger family with a large chest freezer where bulk buying is done on a once-a-month basis. For example, we have pack sizes of 6s, 10s, 24s, 36s and 60s of 'Fish fingers'.

Packs today are much more informative about the ingredients and calorie levels contained in the products. One of the best examples of this is the Ross Weight Watchers range of slimming products on which detailed nutritional information is given on both the ingredients and the calorific content.

From a manufacturer's standpoint, successful marketing of food products is entirely dependent upon our ability to satisfy the preferences of today's consumers, and it is only by studying the trends that I have outlined so far that we can hope to keep abreast of the market and develop products for the future. Already there are some interesting trends emerging about what the consumer in the 80s and the 90s will be looking for.

F. Possible future trends

I would like to take time out and indulge in a little crystal ball gazing about some of the trends that are expected to materialise over the next decade or so.

Let's take, for example, free time. There is no doubt that time spent in formal employment will almost certainly decline throughout the 80s and 90s, and if we extrapolate the current economic and technological impact on society, we could develop a picture which looks like this:

a. Unemployment in the range of three to four million.
b. At least two hours less in the working week.
c. Many more people on a 4 to 4½ day working week, enjoying their shorter working weeks as longer weekends rather than shorter days.
d. Annual holiday entitlement around 30 days or more.
e. Significant number of men aged 55 years and over taking early retirement.
f. The concept of the mid-career 'sabatical' gaining ground among groups other than academics, in particular in arduous occupations amongst long-service employees.

Again if we look at the situation as it exists in Britain at the moment, it is not difficult to conceive of Britain in the 80s and 90s as a nation of 'haves' and 'have-nots', the divides existing in a number of areas such as: employed -v- unemployed; black -v- white ; urban -v- rural; youth -v- not so young; north -v- south; rich -v- poor. Although this all sounds a bit like a self-fulfilling Orwellian nightmare, it is far from an unrealistic scenario and there might well be a situation whereby a food manufacturer is required to produce products that are specific to each segment, a range of products designed for the affluent 'haves' and a range of subsistence products for the 'have nots'.

The very significant changes in the age structure of the British population during the 1980s is also liable to create a number of 'age specific' markets, for example the effective reduction of the youth market because of the decline in the recent birth rate could mean a fall in the market for products such as records, tapes, casual clothes and certain foods. As a corollary to that, there will be the emergence of sales opportunities to old people in many new product categories including food, leisure, cosmetics, health and beauty aids.

The other interesting factor is what some economists have labelled the 'household economy', whereby the home is becoming the centre of work, education, entertainment and leisure. If you think about it, the average level of productive capital in houses today is well above that in the average workshop of pre-war times. We own TVs, cookers, fridges, cars, radios, food mixers, video-tape recorders, central heating systems, and a vast array of other gadgetry and amenities from which we provide a variety of services that were previously obtained and paid for in what we could call the formal economy. This has undermined the commercial viability of diverse enterprises such as spectator sports, launderettes, pubs and cinemas. This is liable to develop even further in the 1990s where consumers may well have the opportunity of bulk buying direct from the manufacturer, thanks to enhanced storage capacity and communications networks integrating consumers and allowing direct contact with manufacturers. Arising directly out of some of these changes is a blurring of the distinction between durable and non-durable goods. Historically, we always thought of durables as things that lasted a long time and carried a big price ticket. As a result of bulk buying, shopping, improved food processing techniques and packaging, increased ownership of household freezers, many food items are now effectively durable purchases, whilst many brown and white goods are virtually non-durable purchases. As affluence spreads and social change proceeds, so traditional essentials such as bread or sugar become 'non-essential', while new products such as mouthwash, hair conditioner, convenient polishes and 'fridge to oven' convenient gourmet foods become 'essential'.

Getting back down to earth again and looking at some of the more predictable trends, I think most people would agree that we are likely to see a continued development of convenience in relation to food. Less formal eating habits, smaller family units and an increasing number of entertainment facilities will all contribute to this trend, creating more demand for products that are designed for individual eating — products such as pizzas, toasted sandwiches, and individual pies. At the same time, I believe that the mundane and messier aspects of everyday cooking will become less and less acceptable to the housewife of the 80s. This is perhaps best illustrated by the enormous impact of products like 'Oven chips' and our recently introduced 'Oven cod', which has effectively eliminated the need for deep fat frying.

The household of the 1980s is already changing direction and I believe we are now seeing a minor revolution in attitudes to food, with traditional cooking becoming much less an everyday event and much more a pleasurable pursuit reserved for special occasions.

Research quite clearly shows that, while sales of convenience frozen foods have increased dramatically in the last few years, there has been an equally strong resurgency in home cooking. This, I believe, reflects the change in emphasis away from everyday meals to cooking for pleasure and is a trend which the frozen food industry must take note of in the future by providing good quality meal components, in addition to convenience foods.

So it would be wrong to conclude that consumers are becoming less discerning. Quite the contrary — I believe consumer awareness of product quality is more keen today than ever, and the food manufacturer cannot afford to ignore this.

While, in many ways, the growth of 'consumerism' has acted to reassure people of product quality in recent years, it has also heightened the level of expectation and increased the demand for safeguards. As a result, there is now more concern about safe products and about the quality of both branded and 'own label' items. In the years ahead this trend will continue and price will become a secondary consideration to perceptions of quality and value. Consumers will demand more facts about ingredients, more 'natural' and 'nutritious' products, with more taste and more information about the goods they buy generally.

The whole area of health, dieting and slimming, has potentially major implications for both manufacturers and retailers. We must meet this demand by providing more informative labelling and by innovative product development.

It is up to the manufacturer to make full use of processing technology and to provide the housewife with products which match her perceptions of quality. To cater for increasing demands for choice, he will have to recognise the development of new 'age-related' markets and the possibility of a polarisation between the 'haves' and the 'have nots'.

G. Conclusion

I believe that the 60s and 70s were two decades where attitudes and lifestyles underwent quite radical changes which have led to a much less formal approach to food and a much greater appreciation of the advantages of convenience. The successful manufacturer of the future will be the one who recognises the trends and has the facilities to meet changing consumer demands, who can maintain novelty and interest through new product development, and can maintain a high standard of quality control. After all, it is the consumer who, at the end of the day, has the last word.

6

Farming and the needs of people

KENNETH BLAXTER

Farming is usually regarded as the industry which is uniquely concerned with meeting the food needs of people: it certainly produces most of the raw materials which are processed to provide items of our diet. Increasingly, however, there has been an extension of the chain of events between the primary production of farm produce and the food items consumed in the home. Thus questions arise about how far the <u>farming industry can respond effectively to the changing needs of ultimate consumers</u>, what are the determinants of farming practices, the cropping and stocking policies adopted on farms and what the overall scale at which the farming industry operates in the UK should be. These are all matters central to a discussion of food and people.

The broad aspects of the history of farming in the United Kingdom during the last two centuries are well known. As the United Kingdom industrialized in the 19th century, farming expanded to meet the food needs of a growing urban and industrial population. Indeed, the source of these new markets for food was the farms of the country for industrialization and urbanization were based on rural depopulation. In the 50 years from 1851 to 1901 the proportion of the working population occupied in agriculture fell from 28 per cent to 12 per cent. It has continued to fall, particularly since the second world war, and farming in the UK now accounts for only 2.7 per cent of our total labour force.

The opening up of the new lands of North America and Australasia in the late 19th century led to a situation in which world food supplies were in excess and in a free trade situation United Kingdom farming could not compete. Farming went into a decline which lasted, with but a slight and short-lived relief from the food production campaign of the first world war, for a half century until the outbreak of the second world war in 1939 (Whetham, 1978).

It was in the late 1930s, and because of the threat of war in Europe, that the relations between farming and the food needs of people became of major important. The safeguarding of food supplies became involved in defence policy. Arguments were adduced at the time between alternatives of storage and increased home production. The then Prime Minister, Neville Chamberlain, in his famous Kettering speech in July 1938, proclaimed that the government would not increase food production at home, stating that this would destroy the purchasing power of overseas suppliers for the industrial goods that Britain could produce, a lower industrial production would result and add further to the massive unemployment of the time. Reduced purchasing power of the population would follow eventually to reduce the market for home-produced food and lead to a worsening of the lot of the farmer. Instead, to meet the threat of war, the government proposed to embark on a storage policy. These arguments adduced by Chamberlain serve to emphasize a real point relating to the relation between farming and people's needs; farming is economically closely related to other industries and overall economic policy determines its scale. Storage, as a major approach to the impending crisis, was only abandoned in March of 1939 when Czechoslovakia was invaded. Then plans were made to establish a food production campaign with a Ministry of Food to control the supply, distribution and prices of food.

In the 1930s there was a further pressure on the government to embark on a food and farming policy arising from the publication in 1936 of Boyd Orr's book *Food, Health and Income*. This work, originally commissioned by the government and then shunned by it, was published by Boyd Orr somewhat in defiance of official attitudes. It showed the relation between the income of families and the nutritional adequacy of their diets. Boyd Orr concluded that four-and-a-half million people in Britain received diets wholly inadequate in every nutritive constituent examined and that a further nine million received diets which were inadequate in at least one respect. Boyd Orr, pointing out the relative costs of health care and the costs of dietary improvement, wrote 'From the point of view of the state, the adoption of a standard of diet lower than the optimum is uneconomic'.

It suffices to state that the food policies adopted during the war owed much to the views expressed by Boyd Orr and these were exemplified by the work of Drummond and Lord Woolton at the Ministry of Food. In his history of social policy during the war, Titmuss (1950) wrote 'What was remarkable about these war-time developments in the provision of school meals, milk and special foods for certain groups in the community was the unanimity of underlying policy . . .'. Certainly, all the indices related to the health of the population showed that the food policy was effective in improving nutritional status and the nutritionally-related health of the people.

6. FARMING AND THE NEEDS OF PEOPLE

A question arises about how far the farming industry should take credit for meeting the need of the people at this time. The Ministry of Food was solely concerned with food control, including procurement and price control. It was sole purchaser of food both from home and overseas. The agricultural departments were concerned with food production, including price control at the farm gate. The situation was, to quote Hammond (1951), that 'while the Minister of Food might state his requirements for home production, the Ministers responsible for agriculture must say how far and in what way those requirements might be supplied'. There is considerable evidence from the history of the period that the ministers responsible for food and those for farming were often in disagreement and that some of the farming policies adopted early in the war were diametrically opposed to food policies (Hammond, 1951). Reasons can be adduced for the reluctance of the agricultural departments to concur wholeheartedly with the views of their counterparts concerned with food. They rightly thought that farmers could not be coerced and they realized that cropping and stocking policies on farms had to be kept in some sort of balance. This was, of course, before modern farm technology had enabled monocultures to be feasible and practical. Additionally, not knowing how long the war might last, the departments were perhaps concerned with the maintenance of breeding flocks and herds so as to allow for a later expansion.

The response of farming to the real needs of the population, as the latter were assessed by the Ministry of Food, was firstly to increase overall production, thereby saving imports of temperate foods and secondly to change commodity balance by reducing those livestock enterprises dependent on imported grain and protein cakes and meals. The instruments employed to elicit the response were those of price control and acreage grants coupled with elements of direction. The extent of the increase in production and the extent of import saving is shown in Table 1 for wheat, the most emotive of all basic foods.

Production of wheat was doubled, partly at the expense of other crops, partly through the cropping of newly ploughed land. The import substitution, however, was over three-fold. To provide a perspective on these events it should be noted that the home production of wheat during the war was well less than 40 per cent of our present output.

The considerable and invaluable response of the farming industry to the need to provide food for the population during war led to the view at its end that the overall level of farming production should be geared to a perceived nutritional need and not left to the vagaries of world

Table 1. *Wheat imports and home-grown production used for milling '000 tons*

Year		Imported	Total milled	Home production
Prewar	1934–8	5031	5537	1651
War	1944	2824	5347	3138
Postwar	1947	4193	5307	1967
Now	1980	2116	4958	8470

prices as it had been in the 1930s. The 1947 Agriculture Act was designed to prevent the industry falling into a state of depression by providing some form of guarantee about the size of the market, but the problem was to define what the size of the market should be, that is, what level of food production should be aimed at. The result of what, no doubt, were lengthy semantic deliberations led to the statement in the foreword to the 1947 Act that its objective was 'to promote a stable and efficient industry capable of producing such part of the nation's food as in the national interest it is desirable to produce in the UK and to produce it at minimum prices, consistently, with proper remuneration and living conditions for farmers and workers in agriculture and with an adequate return on capital invested'. The term 'in the national interest' was no doubt accepted to subsume the meeting of nutritional requirements, but these were not specifically mentioned.

The Act came into force when the Ministry of Food was still the sole purchaser of food and was designed to provide the basis for expansion of home production through a system of price guarantees on individual commodities with production targets for each. During this time, farming policy was related to people's needs by the benign action of the government in determining the price for farm produce. Much of the policy was concerned, however, not with immediate needs but with the establishment of the potential for further expansion of food production. Grants for hill land improvement, lime subsidies, and fertilizer subsidies are examples of this approach. The hill land subsidies necessarily included an element of social policy as well (Winegarten & Acland-Hood, 1978) so to ensure that this economically vulnerable sector was not eroded.

With decontrol in 1954, the same Act was used to oversee the transition to a market economy. By this time world food supply had expanded to create gluts and surpluses with some countries dumping their excess. The government responded to this overproduction in the world by introducing 'standard quantities', that is, they prescribed the amount of commodities, the price of which they would guarantee and, as the years passed, the commitment of the government became one more related to the total cost of farm support to the Exchequer rather than to a national policy concerned with the consumer's food and nutrient needs. Farmers were quick to realise that their total returns were not solely determined by the deficiency payment, but rather by the price they could achieve in the market. This suggests that at least some consumer preference then began to filter back to farming in a direct way though, as we will see later, the ways were, and still are, far from direct. For all consumers, food was plentiful and cheap; their choice was wide and they had, to quote another Prime Minister 'Never had it so good'. The integration of food and agricultural policy, which had been so evident during the war and postwar years, perhaps seemed less relevant in the 1960s than the need to ensure that farming could continue without a massive drain on public funds. Farm and food prices were indeed very different.

Matters changed in the 1970s, for the USA in particular reduced its grain production and diminished its retention of surpluses. Instability of currencies, the problems imposed by the increase in the price of oil by the OPEC, together with the policy adopted by North America on the grain reserves, caused world prices of food to escalate and, understandably, concern was felt about the short-term security of UK supplies. The government, in a White Paper of 1975, reiterated the necessity of further expanding home production (Cmd 6020, 1975). Simultaneously, transitional arrangements were made for the United Kingdom's entry into the European Economic Community and for adherence to its Common Agricultural Policy. To this the United Kingdom is now fully committed.

The Common Agricultural Policy has two elements, firstly market support and secondly structural support. Market support is arranged first to exclude competitors from outside the EEC and secondly to have common agreed pricing for all member countries, with both target prices and lower or intervention prices for commodities. Intervention agencies purchase in the market if prices fall below this intervention price. Structural support provides financial assistance to modernize farms, to pension off ageing farmers and amalgamate their holdings, thus making more economic units, to provide training courses and to subsidise farmers in less favoured areas, which in the UK are those in danger of depopulation (Groves, 1979).

Admission to Europe was welcomed by most farmers at the time, for simple calculation using exchange rates for the pound, showed that prices were higher there than in the UK. The manipulation of the so-called 'Green' currency and the monetary compensatory amounts, that is, the rate at which common community prices are converted into national prices and the measures to prevent speculation in food commodities, did not, however, work in favour of farmers. The government refused to revalue the 'Green' currency for some time, thus benefiting consumers and easing their transition from a regimen of cheap food to the realities of European prices. Farmers benefited little.

We are now fully committed to Europe and Europe as a whole is more than self-sufficient as far as food production is concerned. This is shown in Table 2 where, for most commodities, there are clear structural surpluses. Arguments about the necessity for a member state's self-sufficiency should be irrelevant within the Community. Insistence on UK self-sufficiency within Europe might be regarded as analogous to stating that within the United Kingdom the Soke of Peterborough or the Kingdom of Fife should be self-sufficient in food production. There is, however, no reason to suppose that national

Table 2. *Self sufficiency in the UK and in the nine EEC member states (Self-sufficiency = Domestic production as a percentage of total consumption for all purposes)*

	UK 1981	EEC 1979–80
Wheat	91	113
Barley	133	112
Oats	97	96
Maize	0*	64*
All cereals	96	97
Beef and veal	91	99
Sheep meat	67*	67*
Pig meat	75	103
Poultry meat	99	105
All meat	84	96
Eggs	100	101
Liquid milk	100	109
Butter	57*	119
Cheese	70*	105
Skim milk powder	239	109
Sugar	52*	124
Potatoes	92	101

*Those commodities for which production is 25 per cent or more below consumption.

The UK produces less than 75 per cent of its requirement of apples, pears and tomatoes. It produces 87 per cent of its own cauliflower. Europe is about 95 per cent self-sufficient in vegetables.

objectives have been submerged within the EEC. A number of devices are employed by member states to protect home markets or their farming communities (Marsh, 1977). For our part, we are still concerned about the security of supplies and have to consider elements of risk to our own industry through the completely free access of others to the UK market. Nevertheless, trade in agricultural produce is growing and besides being a food importing country we are now exporting food commodities to Europe and elsewhere in increasing amounts. Currently we export 14 per cent of our wheat production, 27 per cent of the barley crop, 16 per cent of the beef and 17 per cent of the mutton and lamb we produce, not to speak of 40 per cent of our hops and 80 per cent of our whole milk powder production (Cmd 8491, 1982).

Looking back over the recent history of the relation between farming and the needs of people, we can thus discern firstly a direct link between production policies and nutrient need during times of serious food shortage, secondly a period in which policies strived for the provision of plenty with emphasis on the import-saving role of farming and lastly one in which increasing emphasis has been given to farming's competitive place as an industry in the economy as a whole.

The massive increases in food production in the last 40 years have largely been elicited by the manipulation of price and cost. Additionally, the new technologies of farming appear to have created a momentum of their own. Increases in price obviously encourage greater output; decreases in price have a similar effect for if the technical means for increasing output are available farmers will respond to lower prices or higher costs by adopting new techniques thus producing more and so maintaining their incomes. The responsibility for price and cost manipulation has rested with the government and latterly with the Council of Ministers in Europe.

An answer to the question I posed initially about how the farming community responds to consumer needs would thus seem to be 'through the interpretation of those needs by the democratic process of government, rather than through the unfettered operation of market forces'. This is in no way strange or unique, for virtually every farming industry in the world is a managed one. It is perhaps more pertinent to enquire how the government interprets consumer needs in devising farm policies and, indeed, what people demand of the farming industry.

So far we have considered farming and people only in relation to the supply of farm commodities, their total amount and proportional make up. We have not considered attributes of supply which relate to the price and quality of the foods actually purchased or asked how far people's demands for cheap, high-quality food have been reflected in a farming response. In this respect, only a quarter of the food actually consumed comes direct to households from the farm or farm organization with minimal packaging or processing. The largest proportion is consumed after considerable processing by the food industry, and virtually all food passes through the food distribution system. As Sir Frank Engledow and Leonard Amery (1980) put it 'The social and economic distance from the farm gate to the kitchen table has increased and is covered by a large and highly organized food industry.'

The relative sizes of the three industries concerned with food provision are given in Table 3. This shows that all three are of about the same size in terms of the number of people employed in them. Their structures are, however, very different. Farming is a very large industry made up of 296 000 small-scale enterprises and shows very little evidence of monopolistic concentration. Ten manufacturers now account for about one-third of *all* food sales and about half of *all* drink sales, while for many major commodities the top five manufacturers account for 60–90 per cent of the market. The distribution industry used to be similar to the farming industry — a dispersed, small-scale industry — as evidenced by the ubiquitous self-employed grocers' shops.

Table 3. *The components of the food provision system analysed in terms of the labour employed. (Cmd 8491, 1982)*

	'000 persons	
The farming sector	*691*	
No. of farmers		296
No. of farm workers		395
The food industry sector	*635*	
Milling, baking and allied industries		151
Meat, bacon, poultry and fish		129
Milk and milk products		50
Sugar, chocolate and confectionery		80
Fruit and vegetables		54
Edible fats		8
Brewing and malting, soft and other drink		129
Other food products		34
The food distribution sector	*843*	
Wholesale food distribution		222
Retail food distribution		621

Now, with the growth of supermarkets and hypermarkets and a formation of consortia the top nine retailers market 60 per cent of the country's packaged groceries and the top three companies account for 35 per cent of it.

As far as the present price of food to the consumer is concerned, the analysis given by the Minister responsible for both food and farming, Mr Peter Walker, is very relevant (1981). The basic information he used is given in Table 4 and on these and other statistics Mr Walker made two comments. The first was 'It is [the massive increase in productivity of the farming industry] that has allowed agriculture in the United Kingdom to survive'. The second was that 'the price rises for food have stemmed more from the manufacturing stage than from increases in price of primary commodities' and the increase in output of the food manufacturing industry 'was less than a fifth that received in agriculture'. These remarks and the facts themselves show that farming has been successful in keeping down the cost of its products; it is not responsible for the actions of the secondary industries.

As far as the quality of farm produce in the UK is concerned, it must be appreciated that the feedback process, whereby the wishes of millions of consumers are transmitted through food retailers, food wholesalers, food industries, some in parallel, many in series, buyers for those industries, and farm marketing organizations to hundreds of

Table 4. *The economics of the two major components of the UK food provision system. From Walker (1981). The basic data derive from Cmd 8491 (1982) according to the calculations made by the Ministry of Agriculture, Fisheries and Food.*

		1960	1970	1980
Agriculture:				
Gross value added, at 1975 prices	1975 = 100	NA	97	125
Input prices, in real terms[a]	1975 = 100	NA	93	96·5
Output prices, in real terms[a]	1975 = 100	115	96·5	84
Food manufacturing:				
Output volume	1975 = 100	82		106.5
Input (materials and fuel) prices, in real terms[a]	1975 = 100	111		95
Output prices, in real terms[a]	1975 = 100	104		104.5
Retail price of manufactured food:				
In real terms[a]	1975 = 100	94		99

[a]Deflated using the index of total home costs (GDP deflator) — from: National Income and Expenditure: Table 2.6. NA: Not available.

thousands of farmers who take decisions, is likely to have a high coefficient of economic inertia or drag. This is made much worse if farmers have alternative markets for their products and if there is no quality premium for the attributes imparted at the farm level.

There are many instances in which action by the farming industry has not been in the best interests of the secondary processing industries and the consumer. One of the best documented relates to choice of wheat varieties in the mid-seventies (Russell-Eggitt, 1977). The wheat varieties 'Maris Huntsman' and 'Nimrod' were considerable advances on previous ones in terms of their yield capacity. They were taken up by farmers since it was financially rewarding to them to do so. Such is the avidity of the farming community for technical advance that by 1974 these two varieties accounted for 50.6 per cent of the total crop. The varieties, however, were very poor breadmaking wheats and had high α-amylase activity, unlike those — notably the variety 'Capelle' — they replaced. The Home-Grown Cereals Authority, a quasi-governmental organization, and the Millers' Organization introduced a system of classification to include payment for quality and the wheat market is probably no longer vulnerable to such rapid change. Generally, a number of official bodies through exhortation and market advice do much to ensure that actions of farmers accord with demands made by consumers and the food industry. Thus, the Meat and Livestock Commission, financed by a levy on the livestock industry, has done much to improve the quality of the meat supply in terms of attributes of leanness while the Marketing Boards, and particularly the Milk Marketing Boards, have long been concerned with maintenance and improvement of the compositional and microbiological quality of the products which are marketed through them. Additionally, a massive regulatory legislation ensures the safety of the food supply to the consumer. Increasingly, the farm industry is taking cognisance of specific demands made of it by the food industry and the public. With some commodities, notably the frozen vegetable industry, considerable elements of vertical integration are already present.

Even so, there is evidence that not all people are satisfied with the quality of the food which they purchase from retail outlets. Criticisms are made, specifically about the presence in food of various additives, preservatives, artificial flavours and colourings and, more generally, about what may be called the disappearance of 'naturalness' from purchased food. Part of this concern arises from farm practices rather than from those within the food industry, for whether warranted or not, and despite governmental control of the use of chemical additives, some people are worried about the use of pesticides, other agrochemicals and of animal feed additives on farms and the possible presence of their residues in food. An extreme view taken by a few is that only those foods which are the products of organic farming and which have not been subject to any modern processing technology are acceptable items of diet. Less extreme are the views of those who are willing to substitute their time and additional expense for the convenience provided by modern foods. These families bake their own bread, where possible purchase produce direct from farm outlets, pick their own fruit in summertime and inevitably enquire about the farm origin of what they purchase. All these various groups, which eschew the products of our modern food provision system and choose alternatives, do not, however, represent the large mass of the population. The latter for the most part cannot afford to exercise such choice. In their instance it is the action of the government through its regulatory devices that provides safeguards relating to those aspects of food quality concerned with safety and wholesomeness.

Thus, despite a certain and unquantified disenchantment about the food available, the needs of people for an adequate supply of food of good quality and at reasonable cost appear to be catered for through both government policy and events in the market place, however remote the latter may be from the farm itself. People, however, have demands to make of the farming industry other than as a provider of basic commodities and these relate more to the social aspects of farming.

The population of the United Kingdom is largely an urban one. In this respect we are not unique, for our society is not so highly urbanized as are that of Belgium or of The Netherlands. Although most of our population is now several generations removed from the land, there is still a concern for the rural environment and an almost atavistic attachment to the ideas of an idealised rural life. Sir Frank Engledow and Leonard Amery (1980) put the matter very well when they stated 'A highly urbanized economy with a romantic view of its countryside has yet to come to terms with the unpicturesque aspects of an intensive and efficient agriculture'. Farming is the most obvious of our industries, for it is the major user of the land resource, and farming's activities in large measure determine the rural landscape. Hedgerows, copses, ponds, lanes, and picturesque farm buildings are all man-made; were the land left to its own devices the climax vegetation in most of Southern Britain would be of broad-leaved forest. There is no doubt that farming has changed and will continue to change the appearance of the countryside, converting a close landscape into an open one and replacing a diversity of crops and stock by a regional uniformity. There are some who like to see great vistas of growing corn in a treeless landscape; there are far more, it seems, who prefer the romantic image of time past with small fields, untidy hedgerows harbouring wild life, some of which make serious depredation. There is indeed a divergence of views about modern farming practices and the farming use of land as between those other than farmers who live or work or seek access to the countryside and much of the farming community. The very intensification of farming which has resulted in cheap and plentiful raw food materials of uniform and good quality, while it has met one need of people, has thus perhaps ignored another need which is not readily translated into economic terms. There is concern about the monocultures and about the intensive methods of livestock production that have ensured economic survival for the farmer and provided cheap food of uniform and good quality, and this concern no doubt reflects a somewhat deeper need. This need was expressed very well by Dr Martin Haushofer when he spoke about Bavarian farming and part-time farming at a conference on rural resources (Haushofer, 1981). He said 'people wish themselves back in a wholesome world.'

It may well be that, since primary food production in Europe is sufficient to meet Europe's need for food, greater cognisance should be taken of people's wishes in these respects. This is, however, already being done. Much of the Common Agricultural Policy has a social content and is concerned basically with maintaining a rural infra-structure and types of farming which would otherwise, as a result of economic forces, face decline. The marginal hill lands of our own country are cases in point, and so too are the family farm enterprises in France. Equally, constraints are applied to farming through pro-scription, with ends other than economic ones in mind.

Finally, the relation between farming and the needs of people is undoubtedly complex and indirect. The amount and commodity balance of farming's output is determined by the farmer's assessment of the economic return he receives. In this assessment he considers the prices of farm produce and these are almost wholly determined by government. Government is equally concerned with safeguarding the quality and safety of what is produced, sometimes directly, sometimes in an indirect way. Additionally, government has to legislate with the wider aspects of farming in mind, particularly in relation to the problems of the viability of rural communities, the needs of urban people for recreational areas and for access to the countryside and government has to consider the concern of many about the welfare of farm livestock, intensive husbandry practices and other ·aspects of modern farm operation. Expression of the demand exerted by consumers on the farming industry through the classical channels of the marketplace is certainly much attenuated within the complex structures of a modern food provision system. This, nevertheless, still exists, and it is the combination of this demand and the longer-term action of the government that attempts to ensure that farming meets the complex and changing needs of people.

References

(*Denotes general reference)

Blaxter, K. L. (1972): John Boyd Orr: animal experimentation and the human condition. *Annual Report of the Rowett Institute* **38**, 108–115.*
Boyd Orr, J. (1936): *Food, Health and Income*. London: Macmillan.
Cmd 6020 (1975): *Food From our Own Resources*. London: HMSO.
Cmd 8491 (1982). *Annual Review of Agriculture 1982*. London: HMSO.
Engledow, Frank and Amery, L. (1980). *Britain's Future in Farming*. Berkhamstead: Geographical Pub. Ltd.
Groves, C. R. (1979): *An EEC Agricultural Handbook*, 2nd edn. West of Scotland Agricultural College R. & D. Publication No. 6.
Hammond, R. J. (1951): *History of the Second World War: Food, the growth of policy*. London: HMSO.
Haushofer, M. (1981): Developments in German farming and the country-side. In *Rural Response to the Resource Crisis in Europe*. Centre for European Agricultural Studies Association Seminar Paper No. 13, pp. 70–84.
Hutchinson, Sir Joseph (1972). *Farming and Food Supply*. Cambridge: CUP.*
Marsh, J. (1977): *UK Agricultural Policy within the European Community*. Reading: Centre for Agricultural Strategy (Paper 1).
Russell-Eggitt, P. W. (1977): Choosing between crops: aspects that affect the user. *Philosophical Transactions of the Royal Society of London B* **281**, 93–106.
Titmuss, R. M. (1950). *History of the Second World War: Problems of Social Policy*. London: HMSO.
Walker, P. (1981): The future of food. Press Notice, Ministry of Agriculture, Fisheries and Food, December 9th.
Whetham, E. H. (1978): *The Agrarian History of England and Wales. VIII. 1914–1939*. Cambridge: CUP.
Winegarten, A. & Acland-Hood, M. (1978): British agriculture and the 1947 Act. *Journal of the Royal Agricultural Society* **139**, 74–82.

7

Nutrition, catering and the schoolchild

SYLVIA ROBERT-SARGEANT and JULIET R. GRAY

A. History of the school meals service

The origins of the school meals service date back to the 1906 Education (Provision of Meals) Act. This was enacted to ensure that so called 'needy children' would be provided with a meal whilst at school, in order that their education would not suffer. The Act permitted local authorities to provide free meals to some children.

Between 1906 and 1939, the quality of the service fluctuated with changes in government. After 1939, when the whole population was subjected to food rationing, government policy was established to protect the health of schoolchildren, by providing them with a 'nutritionally sound' meal at midday. This policy, detailed in the 1944 Education Act, was enforced in 1945 by the Provision of Milk and Meals Regulations. These regulations imposed for the first time on the local education authorities the statutory obligation to provide a midday meal for all primary and secondary schoolchildren wanting one.

Nutritional guidelines for such meals were laid down by the Department of Education and Science (DES) in 1966. These guidelines stated that the average meal should provide about one third of a child's daily energy needs (880 kcalories) and approximately 42 per cent of the protein needs (29 g). Surveys carried out during the 1970s (Bender *et al.*, 1972; Essex-Cater & Robert-Sargeant, 1975; Bender *et al.*, 1977) showed that, in many cases, the meals failed to reach these nutritional targets.

B. The current situation

The April 1980 Education Act, in effect, removed the statutory obligation to provide a school meal of a defined nutritional standard. Local authorities are now only obliged to provide meals free of charge for children from families receiving supplementary benefit and to make provision for packed meals to be eaten on school premises. Meals may also be provided for other pupils, but the overall aim of the legislation was to reduce local authority spending on school meals by about 50 per cent. It has been up to each local authority, therefore, to decide how best to achieve this reduction and which catering systems should be used. In many cases, particularly in secondary schools, this has led to the introduction of cash cafeteria systems.

C. Provision of school milk

As well as changes in the school meals themselves in recent years, there have been changes in the provision of school milk. Milk was first introduced to schools during the 1930s, when children paid a halfpenny for a third of a pint in the morning and afternoon. This practice was started following the work of Mann (1926) which showed a beneficial effect of milk on the height and weight of children. In 1940, a third of a pint of milk was provided free for young children, and in 1944 this was extended to include all children. In 1968, free milk was withdrawn from secondary schools, and from 1971 was only provided free to children under seven years of age, with the exception of some older children, selected at the discretion of the School Medical Officer. Although there is no evidence of any adverse effect on the health of schoolchildren resulting from the cessation of free school milk, children who had formerly received free school milk have been shown to grow proportionately more than those children who did not receive it (Baker *et al.*, 1980). This was particularly evident in children from families in lower socio-economic groups. More recently there has been an attempt to reintroduce milk into schools and the government is currently offering subsidised milk (the subsidy is derived from the European Economic Community) to all local authorities. This includes whole milk and flavoured semi-skimmed milk.

D. Changes in eating habits

So far, only food and drink consumed at school have been considered. It is important to know *also* how the school meal fits into the context of eating during the rest of the day, *before* any attempt to make statements on the adequacy of children's diet can be made.

In Chapter 3 we have seen how, until fairly recently, food consumption as a whole has been relatively·stable, but that we have now entered a period where the trend is towards change and increasing discontinuities in the consumption of certain foods. There are indications that there is some breakdown in family eating situations and more individual control over food choices than in the past (British Nutrition Foundation, 1981).

It is too early to say what, if any, might be the nutritional implications of such changes. Nonetheless, it could be envisaged that one group which might be particularly affected by change in eating behaviour is the young, especially children of school age. Truswell & Darnton-Hill (1981) cite evidence to suggest that the food habits of adolescents do differ considerably from the rest of the population. At such a time of change, it is appropriate to investigate what children are eating and to consider whether their health is likely to be at risk. Reference has been made to surveys of school meals. There are also some data available on breakfast eating habits. The Kellogg Breakfast Survey, a nationally representative survey of about 6000 homes, was carried out in 1976 (published in 1977), and repeated in 1980 (Table 1). The 1976 survey showed that about 5 per cent of children up to the age of 12 went without breakfast. In older children, between 13 and 20 years of age, this figure increased to 17 per cent. When this survey was repeated in 1980, again about 5 per cent of children under 12 had no breakfast, compared to 10 per cent for 13- to 15-year-olds, and 19 per cent for 16- to 20-year-olds. Thus, both surveys demonstrated that, as children grow older, there is tendency to omit breakfast.

Table 1. *Children not having breakfast.*
(Kelloggs Breakfast Surveys, 1977 and 1981)

	percentage of children	
Age:	*0–12 years*	*13–20 years*
1976	5	17
1980	5	15

E. Eating habits of children today

In order to investigate the eating habits of children throughout the day, a survey was recently sponsored by the National Dairy Council (1982) working closely with the British Nutrition Foundation.

The total sample of 1648 schoolchildren between the ages of 5 and

18 years was representative of the populations of England and Wales (Table 2). Data were collected on 1446 children on weekdays and 302 at weekends. Data were collected on all food and drink items consumed over a 24-hour period — the amounts of food and drink were not recorded. The time of each meal, the point of purchase of food items and with whom the food was eaten were also recorded. The time frame used in this survey is shown in Table 3. The major difference between weekday and weekend timing relates to the morning period at weekends; breakfast and mid-morning snacks were merged as one at the weekends because breakfast tended to be eaten later.

The next section deals with the information from the survey about meals eaten during the weekday at breakfast time, lunch time and in the evening.

Table 2. *National Dairy Council survey England and Wales, spring 1981 (NDC, 1982).*

*Sample number:	1446 (weekdays) 302 (weekends)
*Age range:	5–18 years
*24 hour dietary recall	
*Data collected:	all food and drink consumed (not amounts)
	time of each meal occasion
	point of purchase of food items
	with whom food was eaten

Table 3. *Time periods used in NDC survey*

Weekday		Weekend	
Breakfast	up to 9 am	Breakfast	up to 12.00 noon
Mid-morning	9.01 to 12.00 noon	Lunch	12.01 to 4.00 pm
Lunch	12.01 to 4.00 pm	Evening	4.01 to 12.00 midnight
Evening	4.01 to 12.00 midnight		

1. Breakfast

Almost 90 per cent of the children had something to eat for breakfast. Breakfasts were classified according to five types (Table 4). The most popular breakfast eaten by three children in every five was cereal-based (Table 5). About one child in five had a breakfast based on bread, toast, a roll or crispbread and about 8 per cent of the children had a cooked breakfast. Approximately 13 per cent had nothing to eat

Table 4. *Types of breakfast*

 (i) Cooked — breakfasts which included a cooked item
 (ii) Cereal-based — breakfasts where the main item was cereal/porridge
(iii) Bread-based — breakfasts where the main item was toast, bread or similar
 (iv) Snack — anything else
 (v) Nothing — drink only (not milk drink) or nothing

Table 5. *Proportion of children eating the various types of breakfast*

| | percentage of children | | |
	Total	Boys	Girls
Cooked	8	10	7
Cereal based	57	61	53
Bread based	18	15	20
Snack	5	4	5
Nothing	13	11	15

for breakfast. On average, more boys (71 per cent) than girls (60 per cent) had cereal or cooked breakfasts, and girls were more likely to have had nothing at all (boys 11 per cent, girls 15 per cent).

The pattern varied in different age groups, 67 per cent of the children aged 5 to 10 years had a cereal breakfast, but this had dropped to 47 per cent among children aged 14 to 18 years (Table 6). This age difference was accounted for by small increases in the number having cooked and bread-based breakfasts and by a large increase in those having nothing for breakfast. This increased from 8 per cent in the 5- to 10-year-olds to 20 per cent in 14- to 18-year-olds.

Table 6. *Relationship of age to type of breakfast*

| | Percentage of children | | | |
Size:	All	5–10 years	11–14 years	15–18 years
Cooked	8	6	10	9
Cereal-based	57	67	52	47
Bread-based	18	15	19	20
Snack	5	4	6	5
Nothing	13	8	13	20

2. Mid-morning snack

During the week 35 per cent of the children ate a snack between breakfast and midday which for 9 per cent was in the form of milk. Children in the youngest age group (5–10 years) were most likely to have a mid-morning snack; this may have been due to the higher proportion who had school milk (17 per cent). Most of the 14- to 18-year-old group who missed breakfast did not eat anything mid-morning.

3. Lunch

Nearly half of all children (46 per cent) bought, or were provided with, a school lunch. Of the remainder, 30 per cent brought a packed lunch and 24 per cent either went home or ate lunch elsewhere. Lunch was classified into three types (Table 7). Nearly four out of five children ate a meal of some sort at lunch time (78 per cent). Most of the remainder (16 per cent) ate a snack, which was defined as a single food item, rather than a combination of foods. So, some children were not eating a variety of foods at lunch time. A small number of children (5 per cent) apparently did not eat anything at lunch time. Table 8 shows school lunch uptake in each age group. It can be seen that younger children were more likely than older children to have had a school meal.

For the 46 per cent eating school lunch, food was selected from the categories shown in Table 9. To examine the shift away from the more

Table 7. *Definition of meal, snack and nothing*

'Meal'	— indicated the consumption of a variety of foods
'Snack'	— indicated the consumption of a single food item for example a piece of cheese, packet of crisps, sweets, a piece of fruit, a milk drink
'Nothing'	— indicated the consumption of a drink (not milk drink) or nothing

Table 8. *Relationship of age to school lunch provision*

	Percentage of children			
Age:	All	5–10 years	11–14 years	15–18 years
School lunch	46	52	43	38

Table 9. *Type of school lunch*

The percentage of children receiving the various types of school lunch

One price, set meal	34
One price meal, choices available	23
Cash cafeteria, free choice	24
Not known	18

Table 10. *Meal types*

Type I 'meal' — 'Meals' which included two courses, one course comprising a food such as meats, eggs, cheese or fish accompanied by or combined with vegetables, pasta or rice. The other course could be either a starter such as soup, or a pudding.

Type II 'meal' — 'Meals' which included one course, comprising a food such as meat, eggs, cheese, fish or a substantial snack item such as baked beans accompanied by or combined with vegetables, pasta, rice, or bread.

Table 11. *Type of 'meal' eaten at lunch time according to category of school lunch provided: percentage of children*

	One price set meal	One price meal, choices available	Cash cafeteria, free choice
'Meal' Type I	66	69	34
Type II	19	19	47
'Snack'	10	6	16
'Nothing'	4	6	2

traditional type of meal to a less formal style of eating, meals were classified into two types (Table 10). The most popular type of lunch eaten by children who had a traditional one-price school lunch was a type (I) meal, whereas the cafeteria system offered greater opportunity for the type (II) meal (Table 11).

4. Evening meal

In the evening, 82 per cent of children had a meal, 16 per cent a snack and 2 per cent ate nothing. Of the children eating a meal in the evening, one-third had a type (I) meal and about half had a type (II) or snack meal (Table 12). The older the children, the more likely it was that they had a meal and the less likely that they had only a snack (Table 13).

Table 12. *Type of 'meal' eaten in the evening as a percentage of all evening meal occasions*

	Percentage
Children eating 'meal' —	82
Type I	33
Type II	49

Table 13. *Relationship of age to evening meal consumption*

	Percentage of children			
Age:	All	5–10 years	11–14 years	15–18 years
'Meal' in the evening	82	79	82	85

5. Eating pattern throughout the day

Taking the day as a whole, there were some differences in eating patterns between groups of children of different age, socio-economic group and region, although the regional differences in meal patterns were small.

6. Age

As we have seen already, the distribution of meals throughout the day tended to differ between age groups, with older children tending to eat more towards the latter part of the day, whereas younger children were more likely to have eaten a breakfast and a midday meal.

It is not possible from the data available to know what proportion of the children having nothing for one major meal were amongst those having nothing for the other two meals. We must therefore be careful in interpreting these data. However, the clear finding of somewhat erratic eating behaviour in 14- to 18-year-olds suggests a need for more detailed studies on adolescents. Further investigations would ideally include weighed food intakes and growth measurements and, hence, would permit the assessment of the children's nutritional status, which is not possible from the present observational survey.

7. Socio-economic group

Differences in meal patterns between socio-economic groups were small. Children from all groups appeared, on average, to have a reasonable meal pattern over the whole day (Table 14). There are clear indications from weighed intake data that free school meals may play an important part of the overall diet, particularly in lower socio-economic groups (Cook et al., 1973). This recent survey tends to support that view. Cook and his colleagues showed that the midday meal makes a proportionally greater contribution to the total daily intake, both for energy and for every individual nutrient examined, for children in the lowest socio-economic group. It is possible, therefore, that any reduction in the availability of free school meals, could have an adverse effect on the overall food consumption of some children. Cook stressed, however, the need to know about eating throughout the day, and eating on a day-by-day basis. In order to assess the extent to which possible deficiencies in the midday meal are, or are not, made good during the rest of the day or week, total daily or weekly records of dietary intakes of children are necessary.

Table 14. *Free school meal uptake as a percentage of children who had a school lunch*

	Total	By socio-economic group			
		AB	*C1*	*C2*	*DE*
Received free school meals	17	5	2	11	45
Did not receive free school meals	78	89	93	84	50
Refused to answer	5	6	5	5	5

8. Housewives' working status

The working status of housewives was investigated, to see if it had any major effect on the overall eating habits of children. There was no evidence to suggest that eating patterns were adversely affected by the mother going to work. There were, nevertheless, some differences in the types of meals children ate at different times. For example, fewer children of mothers who worked full time were likely to have a cereal

Table 15. *Relationship of housewife's working status and type of breakfast eaten*

	Percentage of children		
	Housewife in full employment	*Housewife in part-time employment*	*Housewife at home*
Cooked	10	9	7
Cereal-based	50	54	60
Bread-based	20	19	16
'Snack'	4	4	5
'Nothing'	15	14	11

Table 16. *Relationship of housewife's working status and type of lunch eaten*

	Percentage of children		
	Housewife in full employment	*Housewife in part-time employment*	*Housewife at home*
'Meal'	78	79	78
'Snack'	16	17	16
'Nothing'	6	4	6

Table 17. *Relationship of housewife's working status and type of evening meal eaten on weekdays*

	Percentage of children		
	Housewife in full employment	*Housewife in part-time employment*	*Housewife at home*
Type I 'meal'	28	34	34
Type II 'meal'	53	48	49
'Snack'	17	17	15
'Nothing'	2	1	2

breakfast than children whose mothers were at home, but these differences were small (Table 15). The types of meals eaten and the uptake of school lunches were similar amongst children whose mothers worked and those who did not work (Table 16). Similarly, in the evening, about 80 per cent of children in both groups had a meal (Table 17). There were, however, some differences in the type of meal eaten. On weekdays, children whose mothers were at home or worked part-time were more likely to have had a type I meal than children whose mothers worked full time. Despite some differences in the type of meal consumed, children of mothers who worked did not fare worse than children of non-working mothers.

9. Possible conclusions

a. The overall picture of children's eating patterns throughout the day shown by this survey is reassuring, and would suggest that most children in Britain today appear to be well-fed, although quantitative data is needed to confirm this. The majority of children appear to have a reasonable meal pattern — 92 per cent of children surveyed had at least two meals each day. Younger children, in particular, were very unlikely not to have had a reasonable combination of meals during the day. This, however, should not allow for complacency.

b. The present survey demonstrates that the eating habits of 14- to 18-year-old schoolchildren are somewhat erratic. It is recommended that the nutritional status of adolescents be monitored by weighed food intake, and by growth measurements (anthropometric surveys), because there may be implications for the future health of the two million schoolchildren in this age group. It is understood that the Department of Health and Social Security is planning a major survey of this type and currently has a feasibility study under way. If this proves successful, the major survey could then be carried out in the Spring Term of 1983.

c. This survey indicates that the school catering services make a useful contribution to the food consumption of children. Any reductions in this service, for whatever reason, could have an adverse effect on overall food consumption.

d. The major and rapid social and economic changes which have taken place in recent years have been associated with changes in meal patterns and the types of meal consumed. It is likely that there will be further change in the years ahead. It would be prudent, therefore, for this survey to be repeated in a few years' time in order to monitor trends in meal habits. It is hoped that this suggestion will be taken up by the appropriate government departments or by other bodies.

F. Teaching about eating

Nutrition education still has a significant place in the school curriculum. It is essential that nutrition is taught in a practical and commonsense way, starting by teaching about foods that children actually eat. We have seen for many years, sadly, nutrition being taught mainly in a theoretical way, with too much emphasis on the sources and functions of nutrients, accompanied by a mass of data on chemical structures and composition, particularly of vitamins. Detailed studies of scurvy may be fascinating to marine historians, but are somewhat divorced from the everyday decisions that children make about what they will eat and why. There are two main ways in which teaching about eating can be organised. Firstly and traditionally, in the classroom and, secondly, through the school catering service. In the classroom, the aim must be to help healthy children make an informed choice about the food they eat, rather than embarking on concepts of diets for the prevention of specific diseases.

There will ideally be a progression from early teaching in primary schools of facts about food and people, to more advanced concepts in secondary schools' teaching of both home economics and biology. In secondary schools the departments of home economics, which tend to take a more practical approach to teaching, present an ideal main agent for the teaching of nutrition, but there is a need also to develop the nutritional component of the Biology curriculum. Being a practical subject, home economics also offers opportunities for learning outside the classroom which processing units and research laboratories in the food industry could provide. There is also scope closer to the classroom by linking in with the school catering service. It is this second approach to teaching nutrition that is now discussed further.

1. Nutrition education and catering

Whatever is done in the classroom, and however well the information is related to the lifestyle of the child, nutrition is still regarded mainly as a theoretical subject. The school cafeteria offers an opportunity to relate theory to practice, and to consolidate the message that nutritional knowledge and nutritional practice are both important in developing a sound understanding of the way food affects the body and its health.

Since April 1980, Local Education Authorities have adopted a more commercial approach to catering management in schools. It can never become completely commercial in the sense of making a profit, and will be for many years to come primarily a welfare service. Local authorities now have considerable experience in managing cash cafeteria systems and, in most cases, the attitude of the catering manager towards value for money from a nutritional standpoint has been a responsible one.

The child, in free-choice catering systems, has the opportunity of making an individual selection of foods, and not necessarily a wise one. The advent of free-choice systems does offer an ideal opportunity to give guidance and to develop nutrition teaching in a practical and interesting way. One less obvious way this may be achieved might be through a differential pricing system, making it cheaper to eat well nutritionally by using a 'taxing' system on foods. Alternatively, the foods available could be grouped on a nutritional basis so that each child is allowed to select no more than one item from each group. These several possibilities need to be carefully explored and their usefulness in practice carefully monitored.

It must also be appreciated that, more than ever before, the school catering service has to compete with local cafés, home produced packed meals and snacks from kerb-side vans, and this will entail more than simply adjusting the prices to suit the child's pocket — it means marketing. Positive steps can be taken to market the service to its consumers and this in itself demands that the commercial practices currently used in the profit-making sector of the catering industry be used to meet the changed circumstances. Some authorities have already used their press officers in this way and good media coverage has resulted. This initiative could be developed in a number of exciting ways. For example — adolescents and their parents could be informed about other aspects of diet and health. Radio programmes might be arranged to address areas of special concern, for example: current approaches to weight reduction, including putting a proper perspective on some of the fad diets that tend to be popular with adolescents. Is there scope for a regular nutrition spot on local or 'pop' radio stations? There is potential for developments along these lines and those involved in education and catering could usefully explore these areas as possibilities.

The Hotel, Catering and Institutional Management Association has allocated £2500 for the production of publicity material for the school meals service. This will be used by its members involved in catering management in schools to promote the role of the service.

The target groups for this information range from those involved in making decisions at a local administrative level on the future format of the services to local newspapers and radio stations which can help project the continuing importance of school meals to parents in the community. Topics covered in this publicity package could include the nutritional content of meals and snacks, health and safety standards, cost effectiveness of meal production and, no doubt, may also present a strong case for retaining the school meals service. Successful marketing of the school catering service, as mentioned earlier, will also need the identification of customer needs and recognition of the competition in the market place.

2. Fast foods

In the fast food sector, which has developed extensively in the past ten years in this country, customers are predominantly adolescents who seem particularly receptive to this type of eating. Although fast food as a concept is not new, the methods of mass production and standardisation in chains of eating places, which are extensively advertised, is new. Might it be possible to encourage school catering services to consider a closer and more active dialogue with the fast food industry? At the same time, fast food chains could be encouraged to provide salads, fruits or jacket potatoes as an alternative to the predominantly fried foods and sugar-dense desserts which are offered for sale at present. This could be useful to the overall eating pattern of teenagers, especially as the 'family meal is becoming less and less important to the dietary patterns of teenagers' (British Nutrition Foundation, 1981). Is there perhaps a way for fast food chains themselves to intersperse health messages like 'Eat a varied diet' or 'Eat more vegetables and fruit' on their menu display cards?

Similarly, to display attractive eye-catching posters in school canteens, instead of the conventional peg-board menu, might be possible. Speciality promotion weeks, for example, a 'Vegetable week' or a 'Continental week' would also help to maintain interest, as one problem of a cash-cafeteria system is its wide but unchanging choice of foods. Promotion and marketing may sound inappropriate but, with the degree of choice that now occurs at the service counters in school canteens, there is greater scope than ever for such a common feature of a child's everyday experience to be used in nutrition education. What better way to promote healthy eating than in a style that adolescents have already adopted for themselves?

3. Changing needs and practices

Caterers themselves must also learn new techniques if they are to maintain a viable service of high standard and low cost. Training programmes will be needed to initiate staff into new catering methods, particularly when, in the streamlining process, small kitchens are closed and new cook/freeze or cook/chill systems have been introduced into larger central kitchens. Even so, with the high capital and overhead costs which still remain, further efforts may be used to make the school catering service more cost effective, whilst still maintaining its important role as a provider of sound balanced meals for the schoolchild. In some local authorities this is being tackled by increasing the output of each catering unit. After all catering operations in the commercial sector that serve only one meal a day for five days a week for only 38 weeks a year would be hard pushed to remain viable. So, too, in schools' catering. Serving breakfasts, organising and operating morning and afternoon refreshments bars, serving 'latch key' teas before children leave for home, catering for school functions and conferences, or getting involved in providing meals-on-wheels, and supplying food for clubs and evening centres are all possible ways of maximising the efficiency of catering services. Some of these services have already been initiated in some districts and have met with early successes. However, they will need to be assessed in the future when the novelty has worn off and the true costs of the services are evident.

School meals are no longer just a means for ensuring that 'needy children' receive the statutory allowance of protein and energy. The service has evolved into one which can make a significant contribution to the overall needs of the child, both physiologically and academically, and in their social and cultural development.

We are into an era of 'Buying better health' and the school catering service can play an important role during a period of a child's life when they are most vulnerable physically to not getting the nutrients they need.

G. Conclusion

Nutrition education of the schoolchild remains important. Such education needs to relate to the habits and lifestyles of children today. Adolescent schoolchildren (as we have seen from the National Dairy

Council survey) do have somewhat erratic eating patterns. To guide the eating behaviour of children, it is necessary first to recognise present food preferences, prejudices and habits, and these are, to some extent, different in children compared to the rest of the population. This is a time of social and economic change. Thus, changes in eating patterns are likely to continue. There will, therefore, be a need for guidance and, hence, for surveillance.

References

Baker, I. A., Elwood, P. C., Hughes, J., Jones, J., Moore, F. & Sweetnam, P. M. (1980): A randomised controlled trial of the effect of the provision of free school milk on the growth of children. *Journal of Epidemiology and Community Health* 34, 31–34.

Bender, A. E. (1981): Nutrition of schoolchildren. In *Preventive Nutrition and Society*, ed M. R. Turner, pp. 109–119. London: Academic Press.

Bender, A. E., Magee, P. & Nash, A. M. (1972): Survey of school meals. *British Medical Journal* 2, 383–385.

Bender, A. E., Harris, M. C. & Getreuer, A. (1977): Feeding of school children in a London borough. *British Medical Journal* 1, 757–759.

British Nutrition Foundation (1981): *Eating Behaviour and Attitudes to Food, Nutrition and Health*. Report by S. H. M. King. London: J. Walter Thompson Co. Ltd.

Cook, J., Altman, D. G., Moore, D. C. M., Topp, S. G., Holland, W. W. & Elliott, A. (1973): A survey of the nutritional status of schoolchildren. Relation between nutrient intake and socio-economic factors. *British Journal of Preventive Social Medicine* 27, 91–99.

Department of Education and Science (1966): The nutritional standard of school dinners. Circular 3/66. London: HMSO.

Essex-Cater, A. & Robert-Sargeant, S. (1975): Value of school meals. *Health and Social Service Journal* April 5, 758–759.

Kellogg Company of Great Britain Ltd. (1977): *Kellogg Breakfast Survey in Breakfast and the Changing British Lifestyle*. Manchester: Kellogg Company of Great Britain Limited.

Mann, H. C. C. (1926): *Diets for Boys During the School Age*. Medical Research Council Report, No. 105. London: HMSO.

National Dairy Council (1982): *What are Children Eating These Days?* London: National Dairy Council.

Truswell, A. S. & Darnton-Hill, I. (1981): Food habits of adolescents. *Nutrition Reviews* 39, 73–88.

8

Nutrition of the elderly and disabled

BERNARD ISAACS

Animals living in the wild rarely attain the age of their fellows in captivity. As their speed slows and their eyes dim they fail to forage, and die of starvation or are consumed by predators. Ageing human beings do not have quite so grim a struggle for survival, but the foraging system of modern urban life favours the quick and the keen-sighted and disadvantages the elderly and the disabled. The many who are, in addition, socially isolated are vulnerable to nutritional disorders. The processes involved before a hot, nourishing meal finds its way into an elderly stomach can be summarised as: planning; purchasing; preparing; partaking.

PLANNING: involves the *will* to think about meals in advance and *skill* to estimate requirements.

PURCHASING: implies *mobility* to reach the shops, *money* to pay for what is needed, *strength* to find and choose, and *strength* to stand and to carry.

PREPARING: requires *flexibility* to reach high and low shelves, *dexterity* to use tools and open containers, *memory* of time and place, and *control* of sources of power.

PARTAKING: requires *appetite* to want to eat, *mastication* with own teeth or dentures, *swallowing* and *digestion*, and *confidence* in elimination.

If any of these abilities is deficient or absent, the food chain is snapped.

In my childhood, foraging seemed to engage the attention of female members of the household round the clock. Three hot cooked meals were provided daily for the family and were supplemented by snacks of home-made scones and home-made jam. In the absence of motor cars, supermarkets, refrigerators, deep-freezes, dish-washing machines, electric ovens, mixing machines, convenience foods and school dinners, not to mention immersion heaters, metal sinks, plastic bowls and detergents — food preparation, food consumption and food clearance went on continuously. Old people live in the young world

127

where convenience foods are not convenient if they are sold in inaccessible supermarkets, packed in containers which cannot be opened and with instructions which they cannot read.

In British homes there live many thousands of old people whose nutrition is potentially at risk because they are relatively isolated and suffer from disability. Similar difficulties are suffered by the younger disabled. More than one person in 20 in our population is now over the age of 75 years, and probably every reader has a parent or other close relative in this age group. Most are fit and well and function independently, but one-quarter of them are so limited in their mobility by disease or disability that it is very difficult, or impossible, for them to reach a shop alone, while one in ten is totally housebound. One person in ten in this age group cannot see well enough to cook in safety, and a similar number cannot manipulate the controls of a cooker or safely lift pots and pans and their contents on and off a stove. One old person in ten has such severe impairment of memory and concentration as to be a source of danger in the kitchen, either by forgetting to take things off the stove and allowing them to burn out, or by turning on gas taps and failing to light them. One person in twenty is so depressed as a result of loneliness, ill health, isolation and loss as to have no interest in food preparation.

Compounding these medical factors are the social disadvantages of late life. More than one-third of those aged 75 years and over live entirely alone, and most of the others live in a household with only one other old person. Two in every five old people have no living children and another one in five have no children living near enough to enable them to prepare food. Less than one-half of elderly households possess a refrigerator. Those least likely to have one are single women or women who have been widowed for a long time. From this group also come those most likely to have physical and mental disability and to lack supporting family. In addition to all these disadvantages many old people lose their appetite. This is due to a combination of a physiological decline in the sense of taste, diminished energy requirement through lack of exertion, and lack of will to eat because of the loss of the social stimulus that younger people derive from coming together at meal times. The sense of hunger can be allayed by frequent small nonnourishing snacks, which further reduces the motivation to prepare a proper meal. An additional factor becoming more apparent recently is the use by some lonely old people of alcohol as a substitute source of calories.

The picture should not be presented in too gloomy colours. The great majority of old people eat well and keep well, and amongst them are some *cordon bleu* cooks. But a substantial number of the very old, the disabled and the socially isolated do not get enough to eat and need help. It is to the credit of our welfare society that this state of affairs has long been recognised and responded to. First voluntary organisations and now statutory ones as well have established effective and extensive meals services. The target of such services is to ensure that there are no underfed old people in Britain today, but the scale of need so far outdistances the resources that organisations have had to make hard choices. Such choices are becoming commonplace when health and social services have analysed the full potential demand on their resources. All providers of services have to choose between four strategies:

a. To provide more of the same: that is to extend the existing service to a larger proportion of the population at need. This is apparently the simplest process and the demonstration of unsatisfied need can be used to direct more resources to an obviously effective service. However we are now approaching a limit for the use of this method.
b. To maintain the existing level of services and add new recipients only when old ones drop out. This involves the creation of a waiting list, generates widespread dissatisfaction and often ensures that the service reaches those who pull the most strings rather than those whose needs are greatest.
c. To spread the service more thinly and more widely, that is to reduce the level of help given to those already receiving the service and use the released resources to give a similarly low level of service to others. This is a painful and self-defeating exercise akin to pulling a drowning man out of the water and pushing him back in again.
d. To take a hard look at the service and at the resources and redesign it radically and hard-headedly so that help is given only where it is needed and only in the form in which it is required.

The scope for all of these changes is severely limited, but this seems the most promising possibility to explore.

Meals-on-wheels and luncheon clubs have been of inestimable value to countless old people, but transport and other costs are high, and in most areas little expansion is now possible. With the 'wheels' now costing almost as much as the 'meals', should not expansion be concentrated on 'meals-without-wheels'? By 'meals-without-wheels' I mean food (rather than meals) that is brought in to housebound people, or meals that are given to the recipient outside his or her own home. The great majority of these meals are the result of spontaneous family or friendly or neighbourly concern. No charge is made, or at most the recipient pays for the ingredients and no record is kept. But for an unknown number of people the supply of meals has followed some official intervention. The meal may be provided by a home help, or by a neighbour or friend at the instigation of the home help or meals service, and the recipient pays an agreed amount to the provider. The activity may take one of three forms:

a. A 'cook-in', in which the helper comes to the client's home and cooks there.
b. A 'carry-in', in which the helper cooks in her own kitchen, usually while providing a meal for her own family and brings the meal in.
c. An 'eat-out', in which the recipient sits at the helper's table and eats with her family.

I wonder to what extent nutritional deficiency in the elderly, the housebound and the disabled could be improved by developing 'meals-without-wheels'? There is the advantage of the person being given a meal at the most suitable time, and with consideration for personal taste and specific defects. A little low technology helps: for example, many chair-bound old people are sustained at home during the day, while their relatives are out at work, by hot drinks from a vacuum flask. We are still faced with a generation of very old people whose houses are poorly equipped, but their successors should at least have refrigerators with deep-freeze compartments.

In those parts of the country where old people are genuinely integrated into mixed-age communities, 'meals-without-wheels' is probably already an active process and could be further stimulated through the local knowledge of a health visitor or home help. But many old people find themselves living in areas where neighbours are out at work all day and no one is cooking a hot midday meal in the adjacent buildings.

The history of spontaneous services is that they function well until someone comes along to organise them and they then become bureaucratic and cost more than can be afforded so they are cut and disappear entirely. This mistake must be avoided. Maybe the way to develop is to increase the capacity of the meals-on-wheels service to organise 'meals-without-wheels' by providing more investigators to study alternative patterns of delivery of care to individual clients.

Thinking in slogans has, in the past, been our undoing. This dates from the discovery of 'the elderly' as a 'problem', leading to a series of 'solutions', most of which were inappropriate, ineffective or illusory. Community care was invented to describe something that had always been there, and today 'self help' is being proclaimed as the gateway to the brave new world. Malnutrition is the effect of disease much more often than it is the cause of it. Correction and the necessary skill will not come from single solutions. Methods with low organisational costs are likely to make most headway in straitened economic circumstances. 'Meals-without-wheels', slogan though it be, may be one way of thinking about improving the nutrition of the elderly, the disabled and the housebound.

9

Catering with special reference to
the public sector

GEORGE GLEW and ALAN WARD

A. Introduction

'Large scale catering' and 'mass feeding' are terms used to describe the
production and service of food to people outside their own homes, in
factory canteens, in schools and other educational establishments,
hospitals, prisons, in the armed forces and in homes for children, the
disabled, the elderly and other specialised residential groups. The term
'institutional catering' is also used for the majority of these operations,
but this term would not include factory canteens or catering for the
armed forces. In all the above instances, the customary arrangements
whereby a family (including within this term a single person living
alone) provides for its food needs are replaced by services employing
specialised workers, with a scale of operation greater than that of a
normal household. The provision of food and drink is not, however,
the sole or even the primary function of the establishments considered
above. This differentiates them from cafés, restaurants, inns and
public houses and other establishments whose main business is the
provision and sale of food and drink and whose aim is to make a profit
from the enterprise. It is usual to include hotels in this profit-seeking
group, although the preparation and service of food constitute only
part of their main function. The table shows how the catering industry
can be divided into three areas, according to financial aims. Work-place
feeding in commercial firms, together with feeding in private schools and
in private hospitals, appear in the 'indirect profit' category because their
catering activities form part of a commercial operation and make a contribution to that operation, even it, as in virtually all factory and office
canteens, the financial contribution is negative, the service being subsidised.

Most people in the UK make use of the profit sector of the catering
industry for only a minority of meals. As such, these meals do not
affect the overall dietary pattern or nutritional status of such customers

Table. *Categories of catering foodservice operations according to their profit-making characteristics.*

Catering/foodservice industry		
Direct profit	Indirect profit	Non-profit
Hotels	Workplace feeding	Welfare establishments (old
Restaurants	School/college feeding	people, children's homes)
Fast food outlets	Hospital feeding	Armed forces
Takeaways		Prisons
Retail store		Schools/colleges
operations		Hospitals
		Workplace feeding

appreciably. However, the profit sector of catering plays a major part for many consumers in respect of alcohol intake, with consequent potential nutritional problems in relation to obesity and to alcohol-related diseases. This aspect of the links between catering and nutrition is a separate subject, which is not dealt with further here. In many of the institutions in the non-profit sector, a high percentage of the food intake of those served is provided by the caterer. This has especial nutritional significance where the stay within the institution extends over a long period, as in old people's homes, boarding schools and long-stay hospitals. Despite their different objectives, the profit and non-profit sectors of catering have many of the techniques of food preparation and of the equipment used in common, reflecting their common origin in the procedures developed for meal preparation in large households.

In this paper, a brief note is given of the origins of catering and of early attempts to utilise nutritional considerations in meal planning. This is followed by an outline of the present scope of the catering industry in the UK. The practical problems of verifying the benefits, either of the partial provision of meals by a caterer (eg factory canteens, school meals) or of a given standard of catering (eg hospital, old people's homes), are discussed and the modern overall approach to catering given by systems theory is presented. Various of the points raised are then illustrated practically by examples drawn from the work of the Catering Research Unit. This Unit originated in the University of Leeds, but it has recently been transferred to Huddersfield Polytechnic.

B. Historical note

From prehistoric times the preparation of food and drink has been primarily a function of the household. This term, however, covers a multitude of possibilities, varying in scale from a single family, to the extended family, to the slave-maintained rich households of Greece and Rome and to the household of an emperor or a major deity. To take one early example, for which considerable evidence exists, the scale of operation within large households in the Egypt of the Pharoahs was such that specialised workers were required for preparing fish and poultry, for bread making, for brewing and for wine making, as the tomb paintings illustrate. A substantial scale was also required in the kitchens of medieval castles and in monastic establishments of that time, with many tasks now carried out by the food industry still located within the household unit. Gradually those operations of food preparation requiring power and machinery became separated from the kitchen and eventually developed into separate commercial units — flour milling being perhaps the first to follow this path.

As the various institutions came into being in the UK — schools, hospitals, prisons etc. — the methods needed to cook and serve food for the numbers involved were, as noted above, already available. The labour needed was also readily obtained. Some details of meals and diets were recorded at the time and examples have been quoted in Drummond & Wilbraham, 1957. These suggest that in the early 17th century many workhouse diets were fairly satisfactory, being based on bread, cheese, meat and beer. Potatoes and vegetables are also mentioned and, in the north, both skimmed and whole milk. In contrast, school diets at this time were often deficient in fruit, potatoes and other vegetables, giving rise to scurvy. These poor school diets continued into the 19th century. Catering facilities were not needed in prisons, since only bread, and that in limited quantities, was provided so that those who could not secure further food starved.

The 19th century saw many attempts to reduce the cost of feeding in institutions, perhaps especially in workhouses. In the absence of clear concepts of energy needs and of the proportionately higher requirements of children, absurdly low food allowances were often made, with inevitable weight loss in adults and failure to grow in children. Additionally, there were outbreaks of deficiency diseases, such as scurvy and rickets.

The 19th century also saw the initiation of meal provision in factories by enlightened owners, such as the Cadbury, Rowntree, Colman and Lever families (Curtis-Bennett, 1949). For children, the Destitute Children's Dinner Society was founded in 1864 in London and was followed in 1889 by the London School Dinner Association. Even earlier, John Pounds, a cobbler in Portsmouth who died in 1839, dispensed education to children at his workshop and also fed the poor children with hot potatoes and roasted apples (Hawkes, 1884). This is often claimed as the first example of school meal provision for a day school! In America there were parallel developments with the Children's Aid Society of New York serving a meal at lunch time in 1883 and in 1910 the Chicago Board of Education started a meals service.

The 19th century saw the transformation of cooking procedures in the great houses in Britain through the employment of skilled French chefs who had learned from the practices and writings of such outstanding chefs as Carême (Page & Kingsford, 1971). At the same time, restaurants with a high standard were being set up in Paris, using the services of chefs rendered jobless by the French Revolution. Of particular interest for this paper is the career of Alexis Soyer (Page & Kingsford, 1971) who designed and operated, from 1841 on, the kitchens of the Reform Club. He turned his attention, in 1847, to the provision of soup kitchens for the destitute in London, designing a large scale soup boiler for this purpose. This was followed by the setting up in Dublin of a boiler and other facilities for soup making on a scale to serve more than 8000 daily. The equipment included carts to carry soup, which were heated by fires on the carts. These carts supplied further serving points.

Soyer's greatest achievement in institutional catering was his re-organisation of the kitchens and service of food in British military hospitals during the Crimean War (Page & Kingsford, 1971). He has left graphic accounts of the conditions he found in the Crimea and of the steps he took to reform the catering services, from the design of a new stove for use in those hospital kitchens which were inadequately equipped, to the setting out of the method and order of serving the food. Perhaps most important of all was the system for training the soldiers working in the kitchen, who lacked any experience of food preparation. His work was aided by his close association with Florence Nightingale. She said of Soyer's achievement, 'Others have studied cooking for the purpose of gormandising, some for show. But none but he for the purpose of cooking large quantities of food in the most nutritive and economical manner for great quantities of people.' It is worth noting that the rations for the ordinary troops in the Crimea were inadequate, initially in both quantity and quality, but even when the quantity was increased, the vitamin C deficiency was such that many cases of scurvy occurred (Drummond & Wilbraham, 1957).

The perfecting of the *partie* system by Escoffier and the setting up of formal courses for caterers, led in the following period up to the 1950s to a degree of stagnation in significant new developments in catering techniques, although a considerable extension of catering services took place.

The first world war saw the beginnings of a conflict between the government and the advocates of the application of the emerging science of nutrition. The consequences of this are illustrated by Drummond & Wilbraham, 1957, from observations made on the weight and health of boys at Christ's Hospital during and after the 1914–18 war.

In the second world war, the mistaken approaches of the first world war were avoided in Britain, with the nutritional advice of Drummond at the Ministry of Food providing the key to effective planning. The widespread extension of canteens at the work place, of school meals and of provision through the 'British restaurants' for those missed by other catering measures, all provided nutritional support for the system of rationing. The measures taken and viewpoints adopted continued to influence policies in the post-war years, although they became eroded when the Ministry of Food was absorbed into the Ministry of Agriculture and Fisheries in 1955. The combined ministry has indeed given scant consideration to the growing contribution to the national diet of the various forms of catering, nor has it encouraged, so far, research into catering, whether related to nutrition or to any other aspect. However, the retention of the National Food Survey, although it did not take proper account of meals eaten outside the home, ensured that any marked fall in nutritional standards would be quickly picked up.

The work which initiated a fresh look at institutional catering in the UK, in the 1960s, was the survey of hospital catering and its nutritional implications published by Platt, Eddy & Pellett in 1963. The survey included 152 hospitals ranging in size from large city hospitals to some very small cottage hospitals. The best quality and the most nutritionally satisfactory food was that provided in a number of the very small (less than 60 beds) hospitals. In these the cooked food could rapidly be taken from kitchen to wards, the scale of particular cooking operations (eg vegetable cooking) was such that excessive cooking times could be avoided and also supervision was both easily carried out and effective. It appeared virtually impossible to provide really satisfactory food in the larger hospitals. This was attributed in part to defects in the system used, which entailed cooking much of the food some time before the service of a meal, storing the food in hot trolleys in which it was in due course sent to the wards and then served to the patients. The cooking times themselves were often very long owing to the size of the vessels used, so that the cooking of leafy green vegetables took at least 55 minutes in one third of the hospitals, in some much longer. Lack of choice, or choice by the patient only the previous day, together with over-provision from the kitchens, resulted in excessive waste, both plate waste and waste left in the containers. The three groups of staff with responsibilities for patients' food, the catering staff proper who cook and supply it, the nurses who serve it to patients and may also take orders if a choice is provided, and the dietitians and medical staffs concerned with the effect of the food on patients' illnesses and recovery, did not co-ordinate adequately their separate functions. In particular, medical attention concentrated on special diets for particular diseases and medical conditions, but neglected the role of food in the case of ordinary patients who did not have special dietary requirements. The prolonged heating during cooking, storage and transit necessarily involved loss of eating quality but also caused loss and destruction of nutrients, vitamin C in particular. Indeed vitamin C loss could be used as an index of the abuse the food received before reaching the patient.

It was clear that similar adverse effects on food quality would result in any other catering operations, including commercial catering, where food is kept hot for long periods and where it is cooked in scaled-up vessels, used without regard for the increased cooking times this may necessitate. The use of central kitchens in some large cities for the school meals service, from which food is sent out hot to the schools, is one example, while meals-on-wheels, in which a charcoal-heated container keeps food hot during transit from kitchen to the homes served, is a second.

Following the revelations of the Platt, Eddy and Pellett survey, the combined initiatives of the United Leeds Hospitals, which required to formulate plans for catering for a proposed new hospital complex, and of the Procter Department of Food Science, Leeds University, resulted in the setting up of the University's Catering Research Unit in 1966, under G. Glew. Its first task was to attempt to create a system or systems of catering which avoided the defects that had been clearly demonstrated to exist. Financial support for the early work came from the then Ministry of Health and the Nuffield Provincial Hospitals Trust. The section of this paper entitled 'Examples of the systems approach' gives an account of part of the subsequent work of the Unit.

C. Scale of the industry

A report by the Hotel and Catering Industry Training Board (HCITB, 1978) stated that 2.14 million people in the UK were employed in this industry. This figure includes hotel staff not directly concerned with catering. From the Annual Abstract of Statistics (Central Statistical

Office, 1982) it can be derived that about 9.3 per cent of the total labour force in the country is employed in catering and related activities. The industry as a whole had a turnover in 1979 of £8200 million at retail selling prices (Mintel, 1980) and it has been estimated that the total number of people eating out per average week in 1976–1977 was 1.496 million (Self, 1981). Between 1975 and 1979 household expenditure on food per family per week declined from 24.8 per cent to 23.2 per cent of total expenditure. As a percentage of all consumer expenditure per family per week during the same period, meals bought away from home increased from 3.4 per cent to 3.8 per cent (Mintel, 1980). In 1976 it was estimated that eating out accounted for 12 per cent of expenditure on food (Anon, 1978). In 1978 the National Health Service in Britain employed 45 000 catering workers who produced 600 million meals. In the school year 1978–79 the school meals service produced 1103.3 million meals (Mintel, 1980). Similar numbers and trends can be seen from the statistics of other developed countries (Glew, 1980a).

In general, the statistical base for the catering industry is poor and statistics are not normally collected by official bodies. At two recent international conferences, recommendations were made to governments to improve the statistical base for the industry (Anon, 1981; Anon, 1982). The provision of a statistical base, at least comparable with that provided for other major sectors of industry, would help governments to realise the size of the investment that they have in catering, both in human terms and in the extent of facilities used. This could then lead to a greater investment in research studies related to catering which would improve our understanding of the industry, improve its efficiency and enhance the palatability of the food provided while conserving its nutritional status. It needs always to be kept in mind that improvement in the quality of the food to make it more enjoyable and acceptable is itself a nutritional objective, of value even if the nutrient content is the same. But almost always high eating quality and low loss and destruction of nutrients go hand in hand.

D. Assessment of the contribution of catering to health and performance

In a number of studies described by Glew (1980b) it has been shown that the provision of canteen facilities in factories can increase productivity. The same author describes work that suggests that fewer industrial accidents result when workers are fed by their employer.

Most of the studies discussed by Glew took place in less developed parts of the world and the results may not apply in Western countries, where the level of feeding at home may be considerably higher. However, it would not appear unreasonable to assume that hunger-induced fatigue could have an effect on industrial performance.

A major problem occurs when trying to relate the performance of schoolchildren, hospital patients and the elderly to the quantity and quality of food intake. There is no evidence, based on properly planned and evaluated trials, that the consumption of nutritious, well balanced meals in any of these situations leads to better performance. School caterers would like to assume that the provision of a midday meal helps the academic performance of schoolchildren. Nutritious meals, eaten with enjoyment, ought to improve the quality of life of elderly people resident in homes for the elderly and, similarly, such food ought to assist in the recovery of hospital patients. However, there are so many other complex factors contributing to the equation that it is difficult to tease out one factor from another, so that firm conclusions can be drawn on the effect of food provision alone as opposed to that of other factors. Another issue which can crucially affect any evaluation made is the degree of dependence of the recipient on the food provided by the caterer. Any supplementation has to be measured in surveys or trials. Clearly, old people in homes for the elderly are heavily dependent (though not usually totally dependent) on the food provided by the caterer. Similarly, in hospitals for the chronically sick, dependence on the caterer is nearly total, whereas short-stay patients receive food from visiting friends and relatives. In studying the effect of school meals, dependence on the midday meal can vary from highly significant dependence to almost no dependence, depending on the total diet of the child. Furthermore, it would be unwise to assume that low income families necessarily provide their children with a poor diet compared with high income families. The children of high income families may well have a more than adequate energy intake but the balance of other nutrients may be at fault. The food provision in low income families could well be adequate, particularly if the parents are intelligent and show some interest in the food habits of their children. The serious lack of hard scientific evidence for or against the 'usefulness' (measured in terms of performance) of food supplied by large-scale caterers in industrial canteens and by the school meals service, has permitted changes in government and industrial policy with regard to meals provision, stimulated by the drive for savings on the prevailing economies. Because there is no hard evidence for the usefulness of school meals, a government which feels itself hard pressed economically can simply legislate itself out of responsibility for the provision of such a service. The lack of any evidence that food in short-stay hospitals does anything other than keep the patients happy (although, as stated above, this objective should not be despised) leaves hospital caterers at a disadvantage when presenting a case for upgrading or improving catering facilities in competition with the demands of medical colleagues.

Another aspect of evaluating performance relates to the productivity of catering workers themselves. Attempts have been made to relate the numbers of meals produced with numbers of workers involved in their production. Such concepts, which have served manufacturing industry well over a number of years, are difficult to apply to a service industry. In service industries the customer or consumer is a very important and vital part of the equation. It is easy to count the number of meals produced and the number of people who produce them but it is also necessary to measure the extent to which they are actually eaten and the degree of enjoyment which results. A meal not eaten becomes total waste. So a crude measure of productivity in terms of the ratio of output to input becomes less sensible when applied to catering.

The need to take so many factors into account in studies and research in catering has resulted, during the last 15–20 years, in the application of systems theory to catering.

E. The systems concept in large scale catering

Collison & Johnson (1980) have described how general systems theory, which was developed in the 1940s and is now being applied to a variety of activities, may be applied to catering. They conclude that 'The problem in catering, as in many other fields, is that of organising complex activities. Catering involves a complex interaction between food and other materials, people, machinery and money. The Catering Manager has the conflicting demands of the customers, the owners and the catering staff to satisfy, and the views of trade unionists, lawyers, accountants, engineers, food scientists, public health inspectors, nutritionists, architects and a host of other specialists to take into account. General systems theory provides a method by which knowledge from different fields may be integrated'. Cleland & King (1972) have stated that one of the greatest benefits and utilities of the systems concept is the better understanding or perception of complex systems which their use brings about. The need to focus on chains of effects, interdependences, and interrelatedness generally leads to better understanding or a recognition of the areas in which understanding is lacking. This, in turn, can lead to better decisions and, thereby, better management.

The tendency in the past 30 years in large scale catering has been to focus on certain elements of the technical subsystem and ignore the concept that subsystems are interdependent within the overall catering system. In many catering operations within the large-scale sector there is an almost paranoid concentration on the group of activities related to food production. This is largely due to the craft-based education received by many of the catering industry's top managers. The production of food in catering is only one of the many subsystems which go to make a whole system which satisfies all requirements. It might also be said that in the over-concentration of attention on food production there has been overemphasis on the virtues which the use of so-called 'fresh' foods impart. Concentration on one element of the subsystem will inexorably isolate the caterer from the consumer. Large-scale caterers are to some degree protected from the application of market forces by being in the position of having captive customers. However, as subsidies are reduced and government control relaxed, customers will turn to forms of eating which are more in line with what they regard as their requirements. Caterers in school meals, industrial feeding and in hospitals have, in the past, tended to ignore the consumer and to concentrate their activities within the food production subsystem. If this trend continues in the future they may well find that their customers disappear. Those caterers in this sector who have used the systems approach (whether knowingly or not) and have studied the needs of the consumer as one element of this approach, and in consequence adjusted their production processes and products to meet these needs, have seen customer numbers grow rather than fall.

Designing systems

The systems must be designed, above all, to serve the consumer's needs. Consideration must then be given to the best method of serving these needs. There are always constraints of cost, of nutritional requirements, of site and so on, placed up on the planner. Within the defined constraints the system can be designed and clearly will start with the menu (list of foods) that the consumer wishes to eat. Computer-assisted techniques are available which are designed to assist the caterer in defining his consumers' needs (Balintfy, 1980). Having made this decision about needs and, preferably, having tested it, work can proceed on design of the system to meet these needs. The problem becomes one of how to meet the needs within the operating constraints.

An example of the thought which needs to be given to planning the technical aspects of the system is the analysis of how catering labour relates to the degree of use of convenience products. A major factor in relation to convenience products is the value which has been added to them by the food manufacturer. Convenience products cost more because they are at a more advanced state of manufacture into meal components. Hence, less labour is required by the caterer when using them, in comparison with the use of unprepared raw materials. Figure 1 shows this concept in diagrammatic form. The higher the degree of processing provided by the food manufacturer, then the less traditional skills and time are required by the caterer to convert these products into meal components. At the opposite end of the spectrum a much higher degree of technical skill is required from the operatives to convert raw foodstuffs into finished products. Decisions on the degree of convenience or pre-preparation are, therefore, closely linked to the number and level of educational attainment of the workforce. The same example could be used to analyse the system in terms of costs. It would be nonsense to consider the use of a large staff with a high

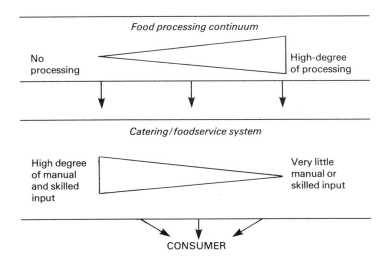

Fig. 1. *Food supply sequence in catering/foodservice industry. (Adapted from Unklesbay et al., 1977)*

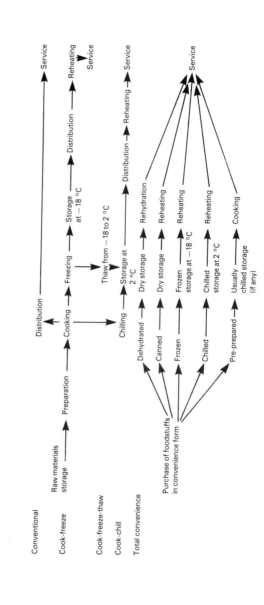

Fig. 2. *Catering systems*

degree of skill in a system which relied exclusively on convenience food products. A further analysis would be to analyse the changes in nutritional quality which result from the use of convenience foods. Such an analysis was completed (Ryley *et al.*, 1978) by the Catering Research Unit in relation to the use of convenience foods in school meals. Figure 2 illustrates another aspect of this problem and shows a number of catering systems and the stages required in the transition from raw material to finished product at the service point. All relevant aspects of these systems have been studied by the Catering Research Unit (see Section F). Unfortunately, practising caterers have often taken sides and tend to support one system of catering or another with great vehemence. This phenomenon again illustrates the adherence of caterers to the production system, to the exclusion of other considerations. The correct approach must be to define the consumer requirements, in which nutritional quality is an essential element, and then match these with one or, more likely, an appropriately chosen mixture of the production systems available.

F. Examples of the systems approach

In its first investigation, to which reference has already been made, the Catering Research Unit was required to supply the Planning Team of the United Leeds Hospitals with data which would enable it to design and install a complete catering system for the rebuilding of Leeds General Infirmary, a 1400 bed teaching hospital (Glew, 1970). Clearly, any radical change from traditional systems required testing on a pilot scale, for which purpose the Hospital for Women, Leeds, was used. This was a 100-bed hospital served by a total staff of about 100. It was located in a separate building and had its own kitchens and catering staff. The compact nature of the building and the modest scale of meal provision needed had enabled the conventional system to operate at a reasonable standard, free of the worst defects of large hospital catering. These defects were the extended time and complexity of kitchen operations needed to prepare all components of a meal, and especially the cooked components, in the run up to a meal time, and the need to transmit the hot food to the wards over long distances in heated trolleys. Although various systems of speeding transit times and of using better designed cooking equipment were considered, it was decided to attempt a more radical solution in order to free the kitchen almost entirely from the link with meal times, and to eliminate the hot transit of the food. The system used (together with related systems which modify it in some respects) has become known as 'cook-freeze'. It allows the kitchens to cook food on a steady, planned, efficient basis, after which the cooked food is frozen in standard packs for storage. It is finally withdrawn from store, transmitted in frozen forms to service points and there reheated and plated.

The many aspects of the system that needed definition, design, study and solution required the services of a particularly versatile research team, the leading members of which, in addition to the Director of the Unit, G. Glew, were a food scientist with household science experience (M. A. Hill), a trained caterer with hospital catering experience (J. F. Armstrong) and a resourceful chemical engineer (R. B. Walker). In addition, there were assistant staff who contributed more than a routine approach to their work.

In accordance with the systems approach, the complete conduct of the investigation, including staff retraining and the installation of equipment to make up the functioning catering system, was set out as a network which was used to control the stages, with the aid of the critical path technique. Various aspects of the system are noted below, with some indication of the results of the work. The new system had to be installed and stocks of frozen food built up while continuing to operate the conventional system, since patient and staff feeding had to continue up to the change over point to the new system.

Consumer response (Glew, 1968). The response of patients to both conventional and cook-freeze food was estimated by surveys, the answers from patients being secured *after* leaving hospital. The acceptability of cook-freeze food demonstrated and also the marked improvement in reactions from patients which a simple choice, made not long before the meal, could achieve.

Nutritional quality (Glew, 1968). The elimination of the effects of the restricted delays in hot transit etc. which occurred with the conventional system in the small hospital used in the trial, together with improved cooking control, gave higher vitamin C and available lysine retention. The results for thiamin and riboflavin retention were unchanged but the losses of these vitamins were almost negligible.

Hygiene (Glew, 1968). The cook-freeze system created no new microbiological hazards, as would be expected. Any hazard is confined to the cooking stages before freezing.

Freezing and reheating. In order to standardise these steps, meal components were frozen in trays with standardised food thicknesses. Reheating was worked out to raise all food temperatures to 80 °C ready for plating after 30 minutes heating in a convection oven. Cooking schedules (Hill & Glew, 1969) were modified to allow for any cooking which occurs in the last stages of reheating.

Recipe formulation (Hill & Glew, 1969). Each meal component was prepared, tested and trials carried out. Starch thickeners required to be selected to withstand freezing without significant texture change in the reheated food.

Kitchen operation. Work in the kitchen was replanned, using work study techniques, to enable steady cooking of components as stock replacements for the deep freeze store. The kitchen operations became less hurried and much more efficient. Staff were readily trained to portion cooked food into six or eight portion trays, to freeze it in the trays and then to remove it for insertion in bags for storage in the deep freeze. Two kitchen staff, with no need for weekend working, were able to prepare as much food as four staff using the conventional system, with much higher utilization also of the equipment.

Storage. The programmes of cooking, etc., were planned to limit storage to one month at $-18\,°C$. This was sufficient to enable the cooking schedules to be efficient, deterioration in store was shown to be of no importance for almost all foods and the size of store required was not increased unnecessarily to allow for long storage.

Food wastage. Plate wastage was reduced, in part due to the new system of choice (see 'Consumer response' above). Overall wastage was very substantially reduced.

Labour relations and costs. It was necessary to avoid any redundancies among staff in order to secure co-operation in the trial, so staffing economies were only possible if staff left voluntarily. It was therefore not possible to make realistic cost comparisons, which would also include allowances related to new capital equipment.

The success of this very comprehensive trial aroused much interest. The Research Unit had to emphasise again and again that future developments elsewhere, which would normally be on a larger scale, required in each instance detailed planning using the systems approach. This would take account of the special circumstances of each development.

The members of staff of the Unit were themselves involved subsequently with further work, briefly described below.

Research and development for the Newcastle Hospitals' Catering Project (120 000 meals per week), which included continuous cooking facilities in a cook-freeze system.

The Leeds School Meals Pilot Study, for 2000 meals daily, which was designed to eliminate hot transit of meals from a central kitchen by using central cooking and freezing and reheating at the schools (Millross *et al.*, 1973). This study included full economic evaluation. It has resulted in a much larger project in Leeds, now supervised by a former member of staff of the unit.

New Leeds Teaching Hospital. The catering for this hospital, the design of which had stimulated the setting up of the Catering Research Unit, is now in operation, using a system based on principles derived from the Unit's work. It is in the charge of a former member of the Unit's staff.

Convenience foods in school meals (Ryley *et al.*, 1978). This study is limited in scope but has demonstrated the nutritional implications of the use of convenience foods.

Meals-on-wheels (Armstrong *et al.*, 1980). This research has included sociological studies of need and has developed more effective techniques for enabling the food to be delivered to the home in good condition, without substantial nutrient losses.

The widespread application and sometimes mis-application of the Unit's work has created some problems for the Unit. Various developments have been, or are being, explored, two of which are the potential uses and dangers of cook-chill systems and the possibility of using central thawing, with chilled transit, to ease reheating in cook-freeze systems. The catering world is currently in the process of change, perhaps without the necessary properly planned changes in human terms at all levels, including in top management, to carry this transformation through most effectively.

G. Education and the future

In case the impression has been given that, having planned a system and implemented it, that is the end of the matter, emphasis must be given to the dynamic state of the catering industry. The solution to a catering problem is static for only a very short time. Allowance must be made for the dynamic state of society, so that change can be introduced and encouraged actively as part of the long-term strategy of the operation. Systems that are incapable of change will die by a slow process of alienation from the customer. Any system must be capable of changing as the customer changes. What is right for one situation in one place at one period of time may be quite wrong in other circumstances and at other times. In order to operate complex systems that are dynamic it is essential that adequate calibre management staff are available and educated to the highest levels. It is not conceivable that a craft-trained operative, without further development, can handle the complex of interrelated problems with which catering management is faced today. We are fortunate in this country in having a number of degree programmes which prepare students for careers which involve coping with the present day complexities of large-scale catering operations, of which nutritional considerations form a part. Existing management must recognise the potential of the young people now emerging from our colleges and allow them to use their skills in an imaginative manner. If this is not done, then the prospects for large-scale catering as an independent, exciting and cost-effective branch of the industry are not very bright and consumers of the end product will be less well served than is potentially possible.

References

Armstrong, J., O'Sullivan, K. & Turner, M. (1980): *The Housebound Elderly — Technical Innovations in Food Service*. Huddersfield: Catering Research Unit.

Anon (1978): Why the world wants quicker meals. *Fast Foods*, Nov 1978, 15.

Anon (1981): *The Role and Application of Food Science and Technology in Industrialised Countries*, ed P. Koivistoinen, R. L. Hall & Y. Malkki. Proceedings of IUFoST/OECD Symposium, Sept 15-17 1981 (VTT Symposium 18, Helsinki).

Anon (1982): In *Symposium on Technological and Economic Aspects of Catering*. Geneva: Committee on Agricultural Problems, Economic Commission for Europe.

Balintfy, J. L. (1980): In *Advances in Catering Technology*, ed G. Glew. London: Applied Science Publishers.

Central Statistical Office (1982): *Annual Abstract of Statistics*. London: HMSO.

Cleland, D. I. & King, W. R. (1972): *Management: a Systems Approach*. New York: McGraw-Hill.

Collison, R. & Johnson, K. (1980): In *Advances in Catering Technology*, ed G. Glew. London: Applied Science Publishers.

Curtis-Bennett, N. (1949): *The Food of the People — the History of Industrial Feeding*. London: Faber and Faber.

Drummond, J. C. & Wilbraham, A. (1957): *The Englishman's Food*. London: Jonathan Cape.

Glew, G. (1968): Attitudes of patients to food in hospitals. *Nutrition, London* **22**, 195.

Glew, G. (1970): Precooked frozen food in hospital catering. *Royal Society of Health Journal* **90**, 139.

Glew, G. (1980a): In *Advances in Catering Technology*, ed G. Glew. London: Applied Science Publishers.

Glew, G. (1980b): The contribution of large-scale feeding operations to nutrition. *World Review of Nutrition and Dietetics* **34**, 1-45.

Hawkes, H. (1884): *Recollections of John Pounds*. London: Williams and Northgate.

HCITB (1978): *Report on Manpower in the Hotel and Catering Industry.* London: Hotel and Catering Industry Training Board.

Hill, M. A. & Glew, G. (1969): The development of recipes for a precooked frozen food catering system for use in hospitals I — General diets. *Nutrition, London* **23**, 68.

Mintel (1980): *Market Intelligence Report.* London: Mintel.

Millross, J., Speht, A., Holdsworth, K. H. & Glew, G. (1973): *The Use of the Cook-Freeze Catering System for School Meals.* Leeds: University of Leeds.

Page, E. B. & Kingsford, P. W. (1971): *The Master Chefs.* London: Edward Arnold.

Platt, B. S., Eddy, T. P. & Pellett, P. L. (1963): *Food in Hospitals.* Oxford: OUP.

Ryley, J., Kleszko, K., Turner, M. & Glew, G. (1978): *A Nutritional Evaluation of Convenience Foods.* Huddersfield: Catering Research Unit.

Self, D. (1981): *The UK Accommodation and Eating-Out Market Trends and Prospects to 1985.* London: Staniland Hall.

Unklesbay, N. F., Maxcy, R. B., Knickrehn, M. E., Stevenson, K. E., Cremer, M. L. & Matthews, M. E. (1977): Food service systems: product flow and microbial quality and safety of foods. *University of Missouri, Columbia, College of Agriculture Experimental Station Research Bulletin* 1018 (March 1977), North Central Regional Research Publication No. 245.

10

Nutrition in hospitals —
the district catering manager's viewpoint

KENNETH LAST

Introduction

Dietary guidelines for health are now well known to many members of
the education, health and catering professions (DHSS, 1978). Putting
these guidelines into effect in a practical commonsense way is difficult,
'. . . not least because people have different nutritional needs, like
different foods, have different eating habits, live different lives and
vary in their susceptibility to disease' (Turner & Gray, 1982). A further
problem is the confusion in people's minds about food, nutrition and
health, fostered by the often incorrect and distorted information
communicated through the mass media. It is against this background
that the hospital caterer has to work, often within tight budgetary
constraints.

It is most important for meals provided to be both appetising and
soundly nutritionally based in order to speed the recovery of patients
and to set a good example, to patients and hospital staff alike, of good
nutrition in practice. To achieve these goals, the caterer needs inputs
from professional nutritionists (eg, dietitians) and support and
encouragement from medical as well as administrative and nursing
staff.

An account is given of the approach adopted in the South Manchester
District by reproducing in its entirety a report prepared by a Working
Group comprising:

Mr K. A. Last, District Catering Manager and Miss E. A. Batty,
Catering Manager (Catering); Professor N. J. Blacklock,
Honorary Consultant in Urology; Dr P. Elton, Senior Registrar in
Community Medicine; Dr J. Leeson, District Community
Physician; Miss E. M. Wilkinson, District Dietitian; Miss R.
Culley, Nursing Officer and Mr H. Seymour, Area Health

Education Officer (Medical); Mr A. Wilding, District Personnel
Officer (Administrative).

The procedures laid down in the report have been adopted in the
South Manchester District.

THE REPORT

A. Preface

The massive improvement in the health of the people of this country
over the past 100 years has coincided with changes in our diet. There is
a considerable body of evidence to support the view that changes in our
diet have been a factor in this improvement. On the other hand, many
of the diseases which now appear to be on the increase in modern
society are being attributed, in part, to the type and quantity of food
that we now consume.

New ideas about the possible harmful influence of many commonly
eaten foods are frequently advanced in the mass media. Much of this
welter of information emanates from the National Health Service
(NHS). While the health service has been in the forefront of
developing and publicising new nutritional ideas, it has not necessarily
been the first to accept this advice and implement it.

The health service, and in particular the hospital and its staff, plays
a well-known part in providing an example of good health practice to
the community.

It is with this background firmly in focus that the District Health
Education Group in South Manchester set up this working group. The
purpose was to produce recommendations on how a greater priority
could be given to the health aspect of a hospital diet. The terms of
reference were to advise on how the provision of food in hospital could
be modified so that 'the content of . . . menus should be such that it is
possible for patients and staff to select a healthy diet'.

In the course of the working group's investigations, it soon became
obvious that a patient can choose a healthy or unhealthy diet from
almost any menu which provides a choice. In view of this, it also
became the intention to recommend a means by which patients and
staff might best be assisted to choose a healthy diet and learn by this
example. Many of the recommendations are based on information
specially collected by the group from three small surveys. This survey
work involved an investigation of hospital menus and also the direct

measurement of what some patients ate. It is hoped that the report, and its recommendations which follow, will provide a firm foundation for future prospects for *catering for health* in South Manchester hospitals.

B. What is a healthy diet?

A major aim of the working group has been to promote the concept and example of a healthy diet through the catering service and the advice given by staff. To this end, it has been necessary to consider what a healthy diet is. Unfortunately, this is not easy or straight-forward. Much of the information with which we are presented seems to conflict. A few years ago, we believed butter was good for us, but now a number of experts say that, if we eat too much, it may help to cause heart disease. People used to be advised to cut down on bread and potatoes because they are 'fattening', but now the advice is to eat more of them instead. Some of the foods we eat are blamed for playing a part in a whole range of disorders including heart disease, obesity, cancer, gall stones, strokes and diabetes.

Besides an increasing preoccupation with health risks, what is responsible for the damage our food may be causing? It is frequently suggested that the major changes in lifestyle in affluent societies are at least in part to blame. Less emphasis on hard physical labour at work, labour saving gadgets in the home, the private care, central heating, and so on, all conspire to reduce dietary energy requirements.

To compensate, we do now eat, on average, less than we used to. Unfortunately, this compensation has not worked quite as well as it should. Although we are eating less, we are not eating less of all foods. We have cut down on some types of food but maintained or increased our consumption of others. (This is not, of course, true of all groups in society. Surveys suggest that some people, such as the old and children in large families may be eating less of some foods than is recommended.) For example, in the last 20 years, the amount of bread and potatoes consumed in the home has halved, but we go on eating the same amounts, or more, of the richer highly flavoured foods, such as meat, cheese, eggs and butter. Less sugar is eaten as jam or straight from the packet, but more is consumed in 'hidden' forms in convenience foods. The end result of this is that the average British diet is pro-portionately higher in fat and sugar and lower in cereals than it used to be.

C. Why do we need to cater for health in hospital?

A question that I am sure will be asked when this report is released for discussion and, indeed, one which the group asked itself is, 'Why do we need to cater for health in hospital?'

Most patients stay for only a comparatively short time in the institution. In a lifetime of poor diet, a few days in hospital is hardly likely to make a great deal of difference. This is not to say that even a short exposure to a healthy diet cannot provide some immediate benefit. Many patients in hospital are probably concerned with such a basic function as going to the toilet. A diet with a reasonably high fibre content can avoid the inconvenience and discomfort of constipation. There is also the minority of patients for whom the hospital does provide long-term care and therefore the staff who spend a considerable period of time in hospital. For these two groups, healthy catering can have some benefit of and by itself.

For many patients, the major benefits of healthy eating are twofold: firstly to allow them to try a healthy diet and get used to it, and secondly to learn, by example and description, what constitutes a healthy diet. Our normal everyday diet is notoriously difficult to change. There are habits and routines of purchasing and cooking which are deeply ingrained. For this reason, information on a healthy diet is, by itself, unlikely to change a family menu.

The advantage of the example provided by healthy hospital catering is that it allows people to try dishes and foods that they might, under normal circumstances, have no chance to sample. It may also allow patients to overcome food prejudices that might otherwise never be confronted. This is not to suggest that all patients consume a poor diet at home. For those who do have a good diet, healthy catering means that they will not have to suffer the dissatisfaction of a less than satisfactory diet during their stay.

With the steady change in medicine and nursing to espouse a more preventive approach to health care, the time is probably right for hospitals to consider more carefully the extent to which they are providing an appropriate educational environment. The success of a healthy catering policy is highly dependent on the extent to which medical, and particularly nursing, staffs are prepared to use the stay in hospital to educate patients.

In 1979, Passmore and his colleagues made an authoritative statement of a prescription for a better British diet (Passmore et al., 1979). In this, they concluded that the diet could be improved by 'moderate reductions in intakes of fat, sugar, meat, and alcohol; increased intake of cereals, potatoes, and other vegetables and fruit; while intakes of milk, eggs and fish, pulses and nuts were to remain unchanged'.

To reverse the trend of increasing fat consumption would, many experts believe, help to reduce the prevalence of heart disease and might also help to prevent the development of certain cancers. Sugar consumption has increased fivefold since 1850, and, on average, we now eat about 2 lb per person per week (almost all is white sugar). Eating this much — it comes to about a sixth of total calorie intake — means that we have to be more careful that other foods we eat provide the proteins, vitamins and minerals needed. A decrease in sugar consumption would probably reduce tooth decay. Some experts also believe that high sugar intake contributes to diabetes and coronary heart disease, but the evidence for this is not conclusive.

Information on good nutrition, the product of the hospital catering system and the hospital staff's own diet are all important in a preventive approach to nutrition. In health education, a valuable commonsense principle is coming to the fore. This principle is that good teachers appear to take their own advice. A preventive service has to incorporate preventive principles into its practice. Its major educators have to retain some consistency and belief in the message that they are transmitting. They must believe in the message to the extent that they themselves live by the principles that they are teaching.

At the level of the institution and the health district, the same principles probably apply. If we are interested in educating the public in healthy nutrition, then we should probably practise what we preach. It is also possible that the community look to the hospital to provide an example of health, although it may be more likely that members of the community can use a poor example provided by the hospital to justify continuing poor health practices.

In summary, the policy of catering for health in hospital has three underlying principles and objectives: —

a. To provide an example of healthy nutrition to individual patients and to the community as a whole.
b. To allow doctors, nurses and other hospital staff to use the hospital catering as a vehicle for nutritional health education with patients.
c. To provide a healthy diet for the immediate health benefit of patients.

D. Problems, methods and procedures

At its inception, the group decided that it would need to take into account two basic requirements in the definition of a policy:

a. What is a healthy diet? The group would need to agree on a prescription for a healthy diet.
b. The group would need to isolate those factors which were most impòrtant in promoting or hindering the provision of a healthy diet. In their deliberations, many factors were considered which might be important in providing a healthy diet. These included:
      i.   Timing of staff and patient meals
     ii.   Range of foods available
    iii.   Nursing routines
     iv.   Methods of delivering food
      v.   Special needs of some patient groups
     vi.   Management constraints of the catering service
    vii.   Cost factors
   viii.   Purchasing policy and cooking methods
     ix.   Requirements of different types of patients
      x.   Consumer views and choices
     xi.   Dietary advice and information

In the course of its work, the task of the group became much less complex. The group concentrated its work on certain specific issues. This is not to say that the issues listed above are not significant, but it was decided that there are three issues which are basic to the provision of a healthy diet in hospital.

These issues which have constituted the major activity of the group are as follows:

a. A description of a reasonable baseline of what should constitute the 'ideal' for a hospital diet.
b. The determination of the extent to which hospital menus do provide patients with the ability to choose the baseline diet outlined above.
c. An investigation of the extent to which patients choose and eat a diet which would conform to the 'baseline' diet.

The work of the group was, therefore, split into these three components. The results of investigations into these issues are reported on the following pages.

E. A baseline prescription for a health diet in hospital

The actions suggested in this report are aimed at the large number of people using the catering service. Catering is a mass service, that is one which, while trying to fulfil the needs of individuals, is a large scale undertaking whose planning and operation must, in the end, take account of an average of the needs of its clients. To do this it needs general or average 'guidelines' on which to operate such as estimated requirements, recommended standard intakes and standard portion size.

In our deliberations it was clearly recognized within the group that catering services, to provide a healthy diet would need a quantitative description of a healthy diet that would suit most people. This sounds a somewhat simpler task than it proved to be. The description of a 'healthy' diet is, as demonstrated in the previous chapter, a contentious and changing phenomenon — changing as new knowledge of benefit or hazard is suggested and/or accepted. There is no simple single generally agreed healthy diet suitable for every individual's health needs.

Our solution to this problem of 'disagreement' between experts was to choose a pragmatic course. This involved taking a comparatively conservative line towards newly promulgated 'dietary health hazards'. We described our baseline healthy diet as one on which, in our judgement, there seemed to be general agreement amongst experts. For example, we did *not* recommend the substitution of poly-unsaturated fats for saturated fats because of the lack of agreement in scientific circles on the health benefit of this action.

The baseline of a healthy diet was of fundamental importance to the work of the group. It was the standard against which the present meals provided by the catering service could be evaluated. It also provided the guide to changes which should be introduced.

The baseline diet summarised in Table 1 and described below, should not be viewed as a precise goal for every individual patient, but rather as a norm or an average of a healthy diet:

Energy content — It is suggested that a diet of 2200 kcalories be provided. The approximate average daily calorie requirements for maintenance of body processes (basal metabolic requirement) are 1500 kcalories for middle-aged men and 1300 kcalories for middle-aged women.

Platt, Eddy & Pellett (1963), in their report 'Food in Hospitals', suggested that the dietary energy requirements of hospital patients should be their basal metabolic requirement multiplied by a diet

Table 1. *Summary of healthy diet baseline (daily intakes)*

Energy (kcal)	Protein		Fat		Carbohydrates		Fibre (g)	Refined sugar
	(g)	(% energy)	(g)	(% energy)	(g)	(% energy)		(% energy)
2200	55g	>10	85g	35	300g	50	30g	<14

factor of 1.8 for recuperative diets or 1.5 for maintenance diets. In their report, 'Recommended Daily Amounts', the DHSS (1979) give average daily energy requirements as 2400 calories for a group of sedentary men (aged 35–64 years) and 2150 calories for a group of women, most occupations (aged 18–54 years). Whilst suggesting a baseline average energy provision, we are aware of the large variations between individuals and recognize the importance of individual energy provision in the hospital situation.

Fat — We recommend that not more than 35 per cent of the total dietary energy requirement should come from fat. There has been a national trend towards a higher percentage of energy being supplied by fat and some reduction of the amount of fat in the diet is necessary. A DHSS report (1974) and the Report of a Joint Working Party of the Royal College of Physicians and the British Cardiac Society (1976) on coronary heart disease have both advised reduction in the total fat in our diet. The second group also advised an increase in polyunsaturated fats. We have not, as yet, recommended an overall increase in polyunsaturated fats, but a margarine high in polyunsaturated fats is available when prescribed.

Starchy Food — We recommend that, as a target, not less than 50 per cent of the dietary energy intake should come from carbohydrate sources, mainly starch.

Sugar — Sugar should contribute less than 14 per cent of the total dietary energy intake.

Protein — Protein should provide not less than 10 per cent of total dietary energy requirement.

Fibre — The daily intake of dietary fibre should be 30 grams. Fibre prevents constipation and is beneficial in treating piles and diverticular disease. Lack of fibre is thought to be involved in the cause of many diseases in the western world. A reduction in fibre intake has occurred along with the decrease in stable starch-containing foods.

This is a highly simplified description of a healthy diet. It was not, however, the intention of the group to rewrite a dietetics handbook but to derive 'targets' on which to base catering practices.

Normal nutritional common sense would be expected to operate within each category to ensure that nutritionally balanced meals were provided. For example, we would not expect that all the protein would be provided by soya beans or the carbohydrates from pasta.

The group were, however, concerned to stress certain qualitative aspects of the composition of a healthy diet. These were:

a. A healthy diet should be presented appetizingly.
b. The food should have a high standard of freshness and palatability.
c. Fresh fruit and vegetables should be a very regular part of the diet.

A healthy diet is, after all, not only one which provides for physiological needs and reduces the risks of illness, but also diet, like health, has its social and psychological connotations. A healthy diet has to provide for these aspects as well!

F. A survey of menus

Once we had decided on a 'baseline' healthy diet, against which to assess the hospital catering system, the next stage was to examine the menus presently provided. In view of the limited resources of the group and the potential scale of this task, it was resolved to restrict the scope of this study. The study was performed on the menus in the three larger hospitals in the District, Withington, Wythenshawe and Christie. Each of these hospitals has a three weekly menu cycle. It was decided to assess the average nutritional content for three days out of this cycle for each hospital. The assessment took account of the protein, fat, carbohydrate and energy content of the standard issues and combined this with the average content of the meals for the three days chosen (a Sunday and two weekdays). The three-day average was based on the average content of each course for each meal over the three days. Table 2 shows the daily average calculated for each of the three hospitals compared with those of the recommended baseline.

In two of the three hospitals the total energy content of the diet was similar to the baseline of 2200 kcalories, and in one of the hospitals, Withington, it was significantly higher at 2700 kcalories.

The relative contributions of fats and carbohydrates were also similar to the baseline, this was again with the exception of Withington which had a diet richer in fat and with a lower contribution from

Table 2. *Comparison of dietary energy intake of hospitals with the baseline*

	Baseline	Wythenshawe	Christie	Withington
Dietary energy, kcal	2200	2324	2243	2742
Protein:				
g	55	82	82	97
% energy	10	14	15	14
Fat:				
g	85	103	94	139
% energy	35	39	38	45
Carbohydrate:				
g	300	254	262	269
% energy	50	48	47	42
Fibre,* g	30	15	14	15
Sugar, % energy	14	24	25	20

*Wholegrain breakfast cereal and bran-enriched bread were both available in the hospitals.

carbohydrate. All the hospital menus had a surfeit of protein (as a contribution to dietary energy), an excess of refined sugar and a low level of fibre. On average, the diets contained about half the level of dietary fibre recommended.

On the whole, this menu analysis shows that the existing menus can provide a nutritious diet similar in energy content to the 'healthy' baseline diet. The general constitution of the diet was similar to the baseline with the exception that protein and sugar made a comparatively large contribution to total energy content, and there was too little dietary fibre.

It seems, from this evaluation, that it is possible to choose a diet which is not too different from the baseline. The next section looks at the extent to which patients choose and eat a healthy diet in hospital.

G. Patient choices and consumption

The purpose of this survey was to look at patients' choices and consumption of the hospital diet. The resources of the group did not permit a large scale analysis of the food consumed. It was, therefore, decided to undertake this work in three wards, one medical and one maternity at Withington Hospital and one orthopaedic ward at Wythenshawe Hospital. The survey consisted of assessing the waste on the plate for each patient against the meal provided. Comparisons of these gave us a measure of patients' consumption. The assessment on the wards took place on seven consecutive days on the orthopaedic ward, four days on the medical ward and three days on the maternity ward. The assessment took account of all the food provided by the hospital catering system, including daily rations of, for example milk, sugar and butter. It did not measure other intakes such as sweets and food brought in by relatives and other visitors.

The assessment gave quite different results from those of the hospital menus survey. Table 3 shows that, generally, the patients in the three wards had a similar pattern of intake. This finding is helpful in suggesting that these results may be more easily generalised to the whole district. The dietary energy intake was most commonly 1000–1500 kcalories per day.

The greatest number of patients within this range were taking 1400–1500 kcalories. The next most popular range of intake was 1500–2000 kcalories, then less than 1000 kcalories, after that over 2000 kcalories. This means that the range of dietary energy which includes the one recommended in our healthy baseline was the one which was *least* likely to be found in these patients.

The energy intake of these patients was low and in some instances extremely low. It must, however, be remembered that these figures include patients who might on some days be very ill.

There were some differences between the hospitals. The daily dietary energy intake of patients in the medical ward at Withington Hospital varied more from day to day than at Wythenshawe Hospital, where each patient tended to maintain a similar energy intake from day to day. This difference may be due to the fact that patients on the orthopaedic ward and maternity ward tended to be longer-stay and/or less 'ill'.

H. Summary of surveys

When it came to analysing the relative contribution of the different components of the diet, there was a fair degree of consistency between the patients at the two hospitals. The percentage contribution to total dietary energy from protein was uniformly higher than the baseline. While the average intake was higher than the baseline, there were some low extremes which could be a cause of concern (22 and 24 grams of protein per day). The absolute weight of protein consumed was not high in relation to the baseline, the high level of protein as a percentage of dietary energy was due to the low level of the total energy intake.

Table 3. *Consumption of major nutrients by patients by patients in three hospitals: average values. Range of values is shown in parentheses.*

	Energy (kcals)	Protein		Fat		Carbohydrates		Fibre	Sugar
		(g)	(%)	(g)	(%)	(g)	(%)	(g)	(%)
Base line:	2220	55	10	85	35	300	50	30	14
Wythenshawe Hospital Orthopaedic Ward									
Day 1: 21 patients	1089	49	18	65	53	109	40	9	14
	(803–1827)	(28–76)		(35–101)		(57–176)			(26)
Day 1: 15 patients	1340	60	17	70	48	182	38	9	13
	(590–2080)	(22–119)		(36–96)		(50–207)			(25)
Day 3: 19 patients	1481	61	16	78	47	151	40	10	10
	(670–2151)	(34–86)		(30–115)		(53–243)			(20)
Day 4: 22 patients	1378	54	15	62	40	133	38	8	10
	(810–2285)	(35–83)		(29–114)		(35–220)			(22)
Day 5: 23 patients	1327	56	16	71	48	122	36	14	11
	(984–2074)	(35–82)		(41–115)		(55–206)			(23)
Day 6: 24 patients	1300	62	18	68	46	121	36	10	11
	(694–2339)	(30–128)		(32–117)		(55–219)			(23)
Day 7: 22 patients	1342	48	16	64	43	135	41	8	11
	(855–1825)	(24–61)		(37–107)		(69–213)			(23)

Withington Maternity Ward									
Day 1/2: 4 patients	1553 (1472–1749)	60 (54–71)	14	80 (64–108)	44	171 (147–210)	42	14	17 (28)
Day 3/4: 2 patients	1467	58 (54–62)	15	72 (68–75)	43	161 (149–172)	42	14	16 (23)
Day 5/6: 83 patients	1297 (850–1548)	52 (41–58)	16	52 (38–60)	37	149 (88–184)	47	11	17 (27)
Withington Medical Ward									
Day 1: 6 patients	1919 (1101–2138)	70 (41–106)	13	98 (55–158)	48	182 (119–296)	48	11	10 (18)
Day 2: 6 patients	1560 (881–1974)	70 (45–91)	15	85 (43–112)	49	142 (80–177)	36	13	5 (15)
Day 3: 6 patients	1623 (1447–1920)	69 (60–75)	17	85 (70–109)	47	146 (103–181)	36	11	14 (23)
Day 4: 6 patients	1151 (971–1575)	55 (34–69)	17	63 (29–97)	45	118 (97–135)	38	12	14 (27)

% = percentage of dietary energy.

Fats, like protein, in absolute weight terms were equivalent to or slightly lower than the recommendation of the baseline. But, again, because of the low level of total dietary energy intake, fat provided an overlarge proportion of total dietary energy. A more detailed analysis of fat in the meals was performed at Withington Hospital. This showed that the contributions of fat from the menu and daily issues (milk and butter) were approximately equal at about 40 g per day. This tends to suggest that fat could be reduced (especially at Withington) by reducing the fat provided through the menu.

The level of carbohydrate in the diet was low (about half the recommended level) and thus the carbohydrate as a percentage of total energy was low as well. Complex carbohydrate intake could be raised by increasing the intake of starchy foods available in the diet, for example bread, potatoes and cereals. One explanation which has been proffered during the study to account for the low energy intake from carbohydrates has been that people still associate starchy food with an unhealthy diet. While in hospital, they take the opportunity to eat what they *believe* to be a 'healthy diet' and, therefore, cut down on their starch intake and imbalance their diet.

Dietary fibre intake was low (intakes varied from one third to half the baseline recommendations). The patients should be able to obtain additional fibre without a radical change in menu. Wholemeal bread and wholegrain cereals could make a very significant contribution.

The sugar provided by the menu was within acceptable limits. It is when the supplementary sugar added to drinks is taken into account that intake is increased to a high level (see Table 3, final column, figures in parentheses).

Taken together, the work from Withington and Wythenshawe Hospitals provides a 'snapshot' of the way that a hospital's diet measured up to the 'baseline healthy diet'. Caution should be exercised with the interpretation of the results. The survey of patients' diet took only a few days into consideration in three wards of two separate hospitals. On the other hand, this report and its recommendations can be fairly said to be based on two pieces of objective research. The validity of the recommendations must benefit from this. The baseline and the two surveys tend to show that it is possible to choose a healthy diet from the existing hospital menus. Daily meal choices from the menus at the three main hospitals have about the same dietary energy value as the baseline of 2200 kcalories. The main divergences from the prescription are a small excess of fat, an excess of sugar and a low level of cereal fibre intake. There is also a small deficiency in starchy food in the daily menu.

A very different picture is presented by the survey of patient choices. It seems that, no matter how well constructed the menu is, patients actually eat a rather poorly balanced daily diet. The average diet is very low in total dietary energy, the most common intake ranging from 1000–1500 kcalories per day. The main reason for this low intake is an excessively low intake of starchy foods. There is also a low intake of cereal fibre. The low starch intake upsets the balance of other constituents of the diet. In consequence, fat and protein provide an overlarge proportion of total daily energy intake. There is also a small excess of fat in the diet consumed which reflects the excess in the menus.

I. Recommendations

At the outset, this report and its recommendations should be read in the light of the group's determination that hospital menus must allow for the variation in the nutritional requirements of individual patients. This is especially true of the total energy needs. It should also be borne in mind that appetite may well be affected to a greater or lesser extent by illness or by treatment procedures. The recommendations which follow should not be viewed as a precise goal for every individual patient, but rather as a norm or an average for a 'healthy diet'.

An adequate diet is essential for health. It is obviously of prime importance to hospital patients. Though it is impossible to give definite requirements of nutrients for individuals, there are recommended intakes for groups. The hospital menu should provide an adequate amount of these essential nutrients. The importance of this provision must be stated first. This report is concerned thereafter with some aspects of a healthy diet which are topical and may involve some changes in hospital menus.

Fats — we recommend that not more than 35 per cent of the total dietary energy requirement should come from fats, in line with national reports which have advised a reduction in the total amount of fat in our diet. In view of differences in expert opinion, we have not, as yet, recommended an overall increase in polyunsaturated fats, but a margarine high in polyunsaturated fat is available when prescribed.

The group recognized the difficulty of reducing fat intake. Fat is an important factor in the palatability of many dishes. Indeed, it is recognised that the aim of reducing fat may be in conflict with the desire to increase the consumption of wholemeal bread. Fat consumption, however, could be reduced by a careful review of cooking techniques and recipes. Lunch-time desserts were viewed as a special target, and we recommend that attention should be paid to lowering the fat content of this part of the meal.

The group also consider, in advance of a detailed examination of the nutritional requirements of more elderly hospital patients, that a palatable brand of margarine should be used in the preparation of sandwiches to contribute to vitamin D intake. In the light of our uncertainty in the present situation, we are satisfied that the reduction in overall fat intake to less than 35 per cent of the total dietary energy requirements should cover most of the health factors of importance that we note to date.

Starchy foods and sugar — We recommend that, as a target, not less than 50 per cent of the energy intake should come from carbohydrate sources, mainly starch. Sugar should contribute less than 14 per cent of the total energy intake.

The amount of staple starch-containing foods has been reduced in this country as in other industrialised countries. In Britain, we eat, on average, about 3½ slices of bread each day. Our target will mean an increase in the present level of starch-containing foods on the menu. The reasons for recommending this increase are to make good the reduction in energy intake due to the reduction of fat and sugar in the diet and because the staple starch-containing foods are sources of nutrients and of dietary fibre.

Sugar is not an essential item in the diet. A high sugar consumption contributes to dental decay and weight problems. There are suggestions that sugar may contribute to diabetes and other illnesses as well.

The main route to an increase in dietary intake should be through improving the uptake of starch-containing foods already offered in hospital menus. The increased consumption of bread is seen as being very important. More wholemeal bread should be provided at mealtimes. Sandwiches, hots dogs and hamburgers could be offered regularly as supper dishes. This might lead to an increase in fat consumption. We, therefore, recommend that this change should be introduced for a trial period on an experimental basis.

Protein — It is not envisaged that there is any need to reduce or increase the dietary protein at present provided by hospital diets and consumed by patients.

Dietary fibre — We recommend an increase in dietary fibre intake. Fibre has a protective role; it increases faecal weight, shortens transit time of food residues and dilutes bowel contents. Fibre prevents constipation and is beneficial in treating piles and diverticular disease.

Lack of fibre is thought to be involved in the cause of many diseases in the western world. A reduction in our dietary fibre intake has occurred along with the decrease in staple starch-containing foods.

There were a number of ways in which the quantity of dietary fibre, particularly cereal fibre, could be increased. The major part of any increase should be in the form of an increased consumption of wholemeal bread. The group consider that *bread should be ordered in the ratio of 2:1 wholemeal to white bread.* In addition, breakfast cereals with a higher fibre content should be ordered in a ratio of 6:1 higher fibre to lower fibre. There are a number of other measures which the group considers to be important in increasing dietary fibre intake, for example the use of wholemeal baps and rolls for hamburgers and hotdogs, the provision of semi-sweet wholemeal biscuits with an evening ('bedtime') drink (the group suggest that wholemeal biscuits should be preferentially ordered in a ratio of 6:1 to lower fibre biscuits) and the inclusion, where it is not detrimental to the taste of the food, of cereal fibre (bran) in some desserts and main dishes. Some experimentation should be undertaken to determine the optimum level of dietary supplementation. Dishes which might tolerate some supplementation of bran might include cottage pie, casseroles, batter and steamed puddings. Wholemeal flour could be used in pastry, sponge mixtures and to thicken sauces.

Despite these recommendations, the major vehicle of dietary fibre in hospital food will remain wholemeal bread. The group felt some concern at the suggestion in the evidence collected that patients may not consume much bread during their stay in hospital. It is imperative that consideration should be given to methods by which people can be assisted to consume bread. Some of these methods have been considered already, including wholemeal bread in supper and lunch dishes such as hamburgers and hotdogs. Some will be mentioned later on in the specific recommendations on staff and patient health education. In general, however, there would seem to be four main avenues for improving the level of consumption of wholemeal bread. These are:

a. Maintenance of the 'freshness' of wholemeal bread: This bread tends to dry out quicker than white bread. The group recommends that there should be improved quality control on deliveries of wholemeal bread. Catering management and staff should take particular care to ensure that this bread is delivered speedily to patients after delivery from the bakery.

b. Improvement of palatability: Measures would include guaranteeing that fresh wholemeal bread and toast is provided in an appetizing form. It was considered important that patients should receive sufficient butter and jam or marmalade. The group is concerned at an unsubstantiated suggestion that some patients in some hospitals may not always receive a ration of butter and jam (and indeed biscuits).

c.   The group recommends that it is important to educate staff and management of the disciplines involved to appreciate the dietary importance of the distribution of butter, jam and biscuits, especially semi-sweet wholemeal biscuits. The group also consider that further work needs to be commissioned to investigate ways of improving the consumption of wholemeal bread in hospital.

d.   Experiments should be undertaken to discover acceptable ways of including wholemeal flour and bread on dishes on the menus.

Health education — The introduction of these recommendations should be co-ordinated to a health education campaign. The campaign would include staff training on the changes suggested. The campaign would aim to involve staff and gain their views on the most effective ways of introducing change. The main objectives of the campaign would be to educate staff, patients and the local community on healthy eating and to ensure that the local community is aware of the example set by the hospitals.

Choice on hospital menus: The recommendations under this heading are of crucial importance in actually assisting patients to choose a healthy diet. No matter what combination of dishes are presented in a menu, what a patient eats is a personal decision — a personal decision that is affected by a great number of influences. Influences such as upbringing, personal taste, presentation on the plate, religious laws, all have a bearing on what a patient will eat. In trying to assist a patient to actually eat a healthy diet, by means of the type of menu presented, the group determined that there are two clear pathways that could be followed:

a.   The development of a system of guided choice whereby menu cards would have suggestions for the choice of healthy diets printed on them.

b.   The presentation of a choice of set menus all of which would be carefully constructed to provide a healthy diet.

The evidence of the limited study commissioned by the group is that a high degree of choice in the menu is not associated with the majority of patients choosing and eating a healthy diet. In terms of existing knowledge of how to introduce changes in behaviour, it is probable that pathway (b) is likely to be most successful. This view is based on the common findings in health education that attitude change does not necessarily lead to behaviour change. On the other hand, changes in actions can lead to changes in attitude. An example of this would be to say that information on the health benefit of dietary fibre may lead to someone associating fibre with health, and to value it as such, but may not lead them to start eating wholemeal bread. On the other hand, wholemeal bread presented on the plate with a meal can lead to a person trying it, getting used to it and in the end learning to accept it as a normal part of their diet.

The development of a system of guided choice, as in (a) above, has the advantage of compromise, compromise between people's desire for choice and the health service's desire to provide an example. The presentation of a choice of set menus, as in (b) above, has the advantage of retaining some choice while creating a greater probability of setting an example which will actually be followed.

On balance, the group find in favour of the presentation of a choice of set menus, all of which would be carefully constructed to provide a healthy diet. As a first stage this system should be introduced for a trial period at Withington hospital. This trial should be carefully monitored to ascertain its effects on patients' diets.

Presentation of food: National criticisms of hospital food which have been found in previous national surveys have related to the presentation of the food — too cold, lacking in colour or taste, lumpy potatoes, gravy and custard are common complaints. It is our belief that a healthy diet is one that is appetising and attractive in presentation. Particular care should be given to neat presentation. Bulk trolley services may offer a particular problem with presentation. The group recommends that the training of all staff involved should be reinforced. Particular attention should be paid to the importance and techniques of food serving. In addition, the importance of nursing staff monitoring, on a day-to-day basis, patients' diets should be a focus for training, and will no doubt be included in the nursing process. The group felt that wards where 'trayed' meals are provided would require extra vigilance.

Fresh fruit and vegetables — Fresh fruit should be more readily available to all patients. Fresh fruit is seen as being particularly important for longstay patients. Care, however, must be taken that fresh fruit is presented in a safe form to geriatric and psychogeriatric patients. In this respect particular attention should be paid to the dental requirements of longstay elderly patients. Dentures should be checked to ensure that they are up to a standard which would allow patients to chew fresh fruit.

The group discussed in detail the relative merits of fresh and frozen vegetables. The decision of the group was that fresh and frozen vegetables both make an important contribution to the diet. Fresh vegetables cannot be defined as healthier than frozen vegetables. A healthy diet, rather, would be better served by attention to the cooking of vegetables in order to maintain their nutritional content, and the provision of raw vegetables and salads.

Ward staff should be encouraged to maintain a careful surveillance of what patients eat. This information should be used as a basis for patient counselling on diet. Health education training and materials should be available to all nursing staff to assist this process. Particular emphasis should be placed on the important role of fibre in the diet in patient health counselling.

Dissemination of this report — This report, with its recommendations, should be disseminated widely within the hospital services throughout the district to medical, nursing, catering, domestic and other staff. Particular attention should be paid to gaining the views of those staff groups most involved with providing catering services.

J. Summary of recommendations

1. The recommendations are not a precise goal for every patient, but a norm or average for all hospital patients.

ENERGY CONTENT

2. A diet of 2200 kcalories should be provided.

FAT

3. Not more than 35 per cent of total dietary energy should come from fat.

4. Fat could be reduced by careful review of cooking techniques. Lunchtime desserts are viewed as a special target for fat reduction.

5. A palatable brand of margarine should be used in the preparation of sandwiches for elderly patients, this would contribute to their vitamin D intake.

STARCHY FOODS AND SUGAR

6. Not less than 50 per cent dietary energy intake should come from carbohydrate sources, mainly starch.

7. Sugar should contribute less than 14 per cent of total dietary energy intake.

8. The main route for increase in dietary intake of carbohydrate is through an increase in foods already offered, most notably wholemeal bread.

9. For a trial period wholemeal bread sandwiches, hot dogs and hamburgers should be offered as supper dishes.

PROTEIN

10. No change in the present amount provided and consumed.

DIETARY FIBRE

11. We recommend an increase in the intake of dietary fibre, particularly cereal fibre.
12. Bread should make the major contribution to the increase in cereal fibre consumption.
13. Bread should be ordered in the ratio of 2:1 wholemeal to white bread.
14. Breakfast cereals with a higher fibre content should be ordered in the ratio of 6:1 to cereals with a lower fibre content.
15. Wholemeal baps and rolls should be used.
16. Semi-sweet wholemeal biscuits should be provided with an evening 'bed-time' drink.
17. Wholemeal biscuits should be preferentially ordered in a ratio of 6:1 to lower fibre biscuits.
18. Cereal bran should be included, where it is not detrimental to the taste, in some desserts and main dishes.

MEASURES TO IMPROVE CONSUMPTION OF WHOLEMEAL BREAD

19. Improved quality controls on deliveries of wholemeal bread.
20. Care to ensure that bread is delivered speedily to patients.
21. Measures to guarantee that wholemeal bread and toast are provided in an appetizing form.
22. Patients should receive sufficient jam and marmalade.
23. Education of staff and management in the importance of the distribution of jam, butter and biscuits.
24. Commissioning of investigations into ways of improving consumption of wholemeal bread.
25. Experiments should be undertaken to discover acceptable ways of including wholemeal bread and flour in dishes on the menus.

CHOICE ON HOSPITAL MENUS

26. There should be a trial introduction, at Withington Hospital, of a choice of set menus constructed to provide a healthy diet.

PRESENTATION OF FOOD

27. Particular importance should be given to attractive presentation of the food.
28. Training of staff involved in the serving of food and also in the monitoring of patients' diets on a daily basis should be reinforced, and will no doubt be included in the nursing process.

FRESH FRUIT AND VEGETABLES

29. Fresh fruit should be more readily available to all patients, but is of particular importance for longstay patients.

30. Where fresh fruit is given to geriatric and psychogeriatric patients, care must be exercised. Attention should be paid to the dental needs of longstay elderly patients, for example the checking of dentures to ensure they are of a standard to allow patients to chew fruit.

31. Both fresh and frozen vegetables make an important contribution to the diet. In the cooking of vegetables it is important that their nutritional value should be maintained.

32. Ward staff should be encouraged to maintain a careful surveillance of patients' diets.

33. To assist in the process of patient health counselling, health education and training, materials should be made available to all nursing staff.

DISSEMINATION OF THIS REPORT

34. This report should be disseminated widely within the hospital services, and particular emphasis should be given to gaining the views of the catering services staff.

Acknowledgements — The group would like to express their particular appreciation for the work of Miss Rosemary Lewis. Without Rosemary's contribution, in the form of a survey of patients' eating behaviour, many of the group's recommendations could not have been made or would have remained unsubstantiated.

Miss Rosemary Lewis was, at the time that this report was being prepared, studying for a BSc in Catering Services at Huddersfield Polytechnic.

References

Department of Health and Social Security (1974): *Diet and Coronary Heart Disease*. Report on Health and Social Subjects No. 7. London: HMSO.

Department of Health and Social Security (1978, revised 1979): *Eating for Health*. London: HMSO.

Department of Health and Social Security (1979): *Recommended Daily Amounts of Food, Energy and Nutrients for Groups*. London: HMSO.

Passmore, R., Hollingsworth, D. & Robertson, J. (1979): *Prescription for a better British Diet. British Medical Journal*, 1, 527-531.

Platt, B. S., Eddy, T. P. & Pellett, P. L. (1963): *Food in Hospitals*. Oxford: OUP.

Royal College of Physicians of London and British Cardiac Society (1976): *Prevention of Coronary Heart Disease. Journal of the Royal College of Physicians*, 10, 213-275.

Turner, M. R. & Gray, J. R. (1982): *Implementation of Dietary Guidelines*. London: The British Nutrition Foundation.

11
Nutrition in hospitals —
the regional catering officer's viewpoint

JOHN RICE

A. National Health Service catering: the problem

Take the Savoy Grill — clientele, waiters and all — and stick it in your average hospital. But, instead of the soignée Grill Room, serve the meals in a hospital ward. And, in place of the elegant furnishings, the lamps, chafing-dishes and hors d'oeuvre trolleys, serve your customers amongst bed-pans, sputum bowls, disinfectant, and much more, and see what happens to their appetite. . . . Now take the same diners and impair their appetite with illness, and surgery, and drugs, and stress, and you're getting near to the problem of feeding patients in hospital, but not yet. . . . Next, get rid of the waiters and replace them with young nurses who love ketchup on their chips and who serve bullet-hard eggs with a cheery smile. Put the ward at the furthest distance from the kitchen and have the whole thing run, not by a restaurant manager, but divided between the supplies man (who buys the food, the bricks, the bandages); the administrator (who decides how much you can spend on food and thinks nutrition is something to do with the third world); a nurse; and a catering manager; and you begin to understand something of the problem of hospital catering and nutrition, without even getting into the field of food production and without even worrying whether patients in hospital should be eating polyunsaturated fats instead of butter; granary bread instead of sliced white; fresh fruit instead of sweet puddings; more vegetable protein; or less salt on their chips, cooked — of course — in soya oil.

1. The market

We are not, obviously, serving that well-heeled lot in the Savoy — well, not all of them. Their culinary backgrounds are very different. Oh yes, we have our share of gourmets (the culinary *cognoscenti*), just as in the community at large, and, like the community at large, we also have our share of punk eaters and fodder freaks, devotees of canned fruit and canned sweetened milk, of fish fingers and sliced white bread. Nor are our patients always prone to accept guidance on the kinds of foods which are good for them. They are not all in hospitals for a short time to repair an accident, or to have a baby — rather less than half are in these categories. But out of every ten patients two are elderly grandmas or grandpas, unlikely to change their eating patterns at the end of a 70–80 year life-span; two are mentally ill; and one is mentally handicapped. It is arguable that for these so-called long-stay patients the catering priority should be more to add enjoyment to their lives, with hospital pubs, coffee shops and restaurants, takeaways, and cream teas; to impart social eating skills to the handicapped and institutionalised, to give them the confidence to eat in the community, and to give a sense of dignity to multiple sclerosis victims by providing facilities for them to make their visitors a snack and a cup of tea, rather than always being the recipients of care. All in all, to put 'heart' into an institution rather than being caught up in the chemicals game of nutrition.

2. The state of play

About one person in six will be a patient in hospital some time this year. Will the feeding be memorable? What chance will they have of good nutrition?

In the three English counties which make up Wessex Region — Dorset, Hampshire and Wiltshire — there will be 20 000 patients in 150 hospitals at any one time, looked after by some 50 000 staff. What chance have the staff of good nutrition? What value does the Regional Health Authority get for the £20 million a year it spends on catering — in patient satisfaction? — in nutrition? How safe, how efficient, how effective are our hospitals in the 1980s?

3. The 'Platt' report

An early shocker of the 1960s, 'Food in Hospitals', a study of the Nuffield Hospitals Trust, by Platt, Eddy & Pellett, gave an alarming picture of the nutritional hazards of being a patient. In case studies in 152 hospitals, it was revealed that only 55 to 60 per cent of the food offered was eaten by patients; that delays between preparing, cooking and serving food led sometimes to the complete loss of vitamin C in potatoes and up to 75 per cent loss in green vegetables. There was a lack of variety and poor quality food, particularly in long-stay hospitals, leading to patients relying on visitors to bring food, particularly for breakfast. (This was a point highlighted some 20 years earlier by the late Sir Jack Drummond and King Edward's Hospital Fund for London, which led to some of the earliest guidance by the Fund on General hospital diets.) All in all, it was a hard-hitting report which, in its recommendations, called for doctors and dietitians to be much more involved in *general* patient nutrition rather than concentrating on the more interesting *specialised* diets.

4. Twenty years on

Twenty years on and much has been done. The best of hospitals have selective menus, meals cooked at the last minute in small batches and whipped off to the bedside in minutes. Patients can choose from a variety of snack or traditional meals up to three times a day, to suit their own eating pattern and particular appetite at the time, and there is a 24-hour menu for patients who are sickly and can't be tempted from the normal menu. There are special children's menus and 'pub' snacks, such as ploughman's lunches and paté on toast. In some long-stay hospitals patients can choose a 'traditional' afternoon tea or strawberry tea in place of the later evening meal, and they can have a beer and a snack as they might at home or at their local, had they the chance. Vegetables are no longer overcooked, but served *al dente*. Staff too can choose from salad bars or grill rooms, or can just go straight to the cafeteria or coffee shop. Some can have a relaxing glass of wine after the stresses of the ward, so that they can enjoy their meals more easily.

5. New problems with improvements

That's the best hospitals. But what of the others — they are certainly not all in that league? And what of the new problems which come with 'improvements'? Yes, many hospitals do offer selective menus, but they expect patients to know what they want two to three days before they are due to eat! In many cases, nurses appear to serve new patients with the selection of the previous patient for the first two or three days until their own choice arrives! And, so often, those plans to provide a centrally-plated tray service to allow nurses time to actually monitor what patients eat has resulted in them going off for their own lunch instead.

6. Shortage of money

Low funding for hospital meals and inflation has meant that many hospitals have cut out cooked breakfasts for patients to save money and in some cases, as in the 1960s, relatives are again bringing in the odd egg — *plus ca change*! With the cut-backs come all those nasty institutional tricks — canned tomatoes instead of fresh, powdered potatoes, roasts sliced wafer thin for economy and stuck in gravy, and spam featured again as the salad alternative — *sans* vinaigrette, *sans* blue cheese dressing, *sans* anything. All guaranteed to ensure that food is left on the plate, nutrients and all. Not a lot of sense in saving a few bob on provisions if it is going to cost you another day whilst the patient recovers strength. . . .

Shortage of money may also be affecting staff nutrition. Traditionally, in the National Health Service, staff eat better than patients — probably the only organisation outside of the prison service where their customers get second best — but continuing Government pressure to mark up the price of staff meals to cover the cost of food, VAT and a proportion of overheads, makes it likely that staff will spend less on food as inflation makes it more expensive and wages continue to be pegged.

And what of Platt's other main recommendations — that every hospital should have one person responsible for all aspects of catering: the production, the service, the administration — not much headway there! Currently nine departments have a finger in the catering service pie — eight of them as a second 'day-job'. Or the recommendation that medical, nursing and dietetic staff should be far more involved in general patient nutrition, rather than restricting themselves to more interesting diet categories. There is not too much evidence of this in the catering manager's battle with administrators to retain the option of the cooked breakfast. The 'let them eat Ready-Brek' lobby was indeed led by the medical staff anxious for a share of the savings.

B. Have things improved?

Well, we hope so, but to what extent? We just don't know. We don't have Her Majesty's Inspectors as they do in schools — or Ronays or Good Food Guides (well, rarely), or Platt-type surveys to tell us. We are in the dark. Certainly our own studies since 1974 have shown that many of the criticisms made by Platt still apply and that the indicator of bad nutrition identified in the Nuffield Report — waste — is still around the 30 per cent mark.'In 1975, the first of our investigations of feeding standards, we identified shortcomings in a cross-section of hospitals throughout the Region and, with the King's Fund, produced guidance booklets showing how to improve cooking, menus and ward service. We also prepared a food quality audit which managers could use to assess their performance and to show patient satisfaction levels. In 1977 to 1979 we reviewed all the hospitals in the Region in a comprehensive monitoring programme covering food quality, patient satisfaction, hygiene, waste, and more. As in 1975, there was seen to be considerable variation between hospitals. And many of the defects identified in 1975 — and indeed by Platt — were still with us.

C. What can a region do . . .?

We cannot instruct hospitals or Districts. Under the latest 'Patients first' NHS reorganisation, Districts and hospitals continue to do their own thing. What we can do is to show hospitals and Districts what the Regional Health Authorities expectations are, how they perform against these expectations, and provide the incentives to improve. Some of our efforts are as follows.

1. For patient nutrition

a. We can identify the indicators of whether or not nutrition is adequate: spending on food; waste levels; patient satisfaction levels taking note of ethnic groups, care groups, diet groups, and age groups; nutritional status; intake levels.

b. We can get procedures to be followed in order to safeguard good nutrition: patient satisfaction safeguards; nutrition safeguards; eating for health standards.

c. We can measure performance against standards and procedures and giving each a statistical rating: percentage of satisfaction achieved; percentage of food wasted; cost of waste per head; percentage of each care group provided with the desired intake level.

d. The performance of 'good nutrition hospitals' can be recognised by giving them some kind of regional accreditation along the American lines and, in so doing, identifying those hospitals which are sub-standard and indicating patients at risk. In Wessex, shall we recognise an accredited hospital with a single star rating and hospitals which perform better up to four star ratings depending upon the proportion of the desired standards being applied, for even higher levels of patient satisfaction and nutrition.

e. We can identify a *supremo* within each hospital, who shall be responsible for co-ordinating the nine disciplines involved in the catering service to patients; to achieve standards required, and to agree programmes and timetables to overcome the shortcomings to get the hospital accredited. The hospital administrator will be the *supremo* responsible to the district administrator on how that hospital performs and will be able to call upon the district specialist advisers in catering, medicine, dietetics, nursing, or whatever to help him achieve that goal.

2. For staff nutrition

Patients must, of course, get the priority because it is they we are in the business of serving. Next year we shall be designing a staff nutrition review. In this case, our risk categories may well be night staff, staff working long hours, the lowest paid, or those with a high sickness record.

D. Conclusions

a. Good nutrition is giving patients what they want — and listing 'healthy' foods for them to choose from.
b. Good nutrition requires high quality and soignée — caring — catering.
c. More money will be needed — but savings can be made. These *must* be identified and proven before improvements are possible.
d. The first step to good nutrition is to get rid of bureaucratic lunacies.
e. Health Authorities must help by pressurising hospitals to achieve good nutrition.

References

Platt, B. S., Eddy, T. P. & Pellett, P. L. (1963): *Food in Hospitals*. A report of the Nuffield Provincial Hospitals Trust. Oxford: OUP.
Wessex Health Authority (1975): *Better Food for Patients*. London: King Edward's Hospital Fund for London. (This book is accompanied by the guidance books mentioned in the text.)

Index